The Wild Child

Mary Jo Putney

The Wild Child

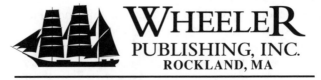

WHEELER
PUBLISHING, INC.
ROCKLAND, MA

★ AN AMERICAN COMPANY ★

Published in Large Print by arrangement with The Ballantine Publishing Group, a division of Random House, Inc., in the United States and Canada.

Wheeler Large Print Book Series.

Set in 16 pt Plantin.

Library of Congress Cataloging-in-Publication Data

Putney, Mary Jo.
    The wild child / Mary Jo Putney.
        p. (large print) cm.(Wheeler large print book series)
    ISBN 1-56895-790-4 (hardcover)
    1. Twins—Fiction. 2. Brothers—Fiction. 3. England—Fiction
4. Large type books.
I. Title. II. Series
[PS3566.U83W55   1999b]
813'.54—dc21   99-048205 CIP

To libraries and librarians:
God bless you, every one

I met a lady in the meads
Full beautiful, a faery's child.
Her hair was long, her foot was light,
and her eyes were wild.

　　　—John Keats,
　　　"La Belle Dame Sans Merci"

Prologue

As the two men climbed the steps inside Grillon's Hotel, the slighter one pushed ahead impatiently. His taller companion touched his arm in warning. "This can't be the right girl, Amworth."

"Of course it's Meriel," Lord Amworth retorted. "How many lost blond English girls can there be in northern India?"

The lines in Lord Grahame's harshly weathered face deepened. "I saw the ruins at Alwari when they were still smoking, Amworth. No one, much less a five-year-old child, could have survived the massacre and fire."

The other man frowned. "We'll know soon enough."

They reached the upper hall and walked to the room where the newly arrived party was staying. One sharp knock and a plump, elderly woman admitted them. "I'm Mrs. Madison, your lordships. Good of you to come so quickly."

"And it was very good of you to accompany the child back from India, Mrs. Madison." Grahame's restless gaze scanned the receiving room. "Where is the girl?"

"In the bedroom, my lord." Mrs. Madison gestured.

They crossed the sitting room and looked through the open door. On the bed, a small, fragile girl was solemnly arranging cut flowers in an arc in front of her, a cascade of hair so

1

pale it was almost white falling about her face. She glanced up, revealing elfin features and widely spaced eyes. There was only the faintest flicker in the pale green depths before she dropped her gaze to the flowers again.

"Such a pity what happened to her, but she's never a bit of trouble," Mrs. Madison volunteered. "Is she your niece?"

Amworth exclaimed, "It's Meriel! She's the image of my sister at that age." He dropped on one knee by the bed. "Meriel, do you remember me? Your uncle Oliver?"

She ignored him totally. He glanced at Mrs. Madison. "Has she become deaf?"

"Not deaf, but her wits are gone, destroyed by the horrors of her captivity. The physicians who examined her in India said she'd always be a child."

"Maybe she'll recognize me. She was only an infant when her parents left England, but she knew me when she was five." Grahame also knelt within the girl's line of sight. Taking one tiny hand, he said intensely, "Meriel, it's your uncle Francis, your father's brother. Remember the pony rides in the garden at Cambay?"

She pulled her hand away as if he didn't exist and carefully placed a lily next to a yellow rose. Apparently she was sorting the blooms by color and size. Grahame exhaled roughly. "She's always like this?"

"She notices Kamal a bit, but no one else. She just lives in her own world." Mrs. Madison nodded toward the corner of the room, where a turbaned and bearded young Indian watched in silence. When the English lords looked in his direction, he pressed his hands together in front of his chest and bowed, but he was as silent as Meriel.

In a whisper that penetrated more thoroughly than a regular voice, Mrs. Madison explained, "He's a eunuch, you know. A harem guard. The maharajah chose him to escort Lady Meriel to Cambay. Since she didn't want to be separated from the fellow, it was decided to bring him to England. Very useful he's been, too."

Looking shaken, Lord Amworth allowed himself to be guided back to the sitting room by Lord Grahame. "Dear God, what a tragedy! She was such a bright, sweet child. Her parents doted on her. Perhaps...perhaps someday she might regain her wits."

"It's been over two years since her parents died, the better part of a year since she was returned to English hands. If she were going to recover, surely there would be some sign by now." Grahame's face was almost as pale as Amworth's. "An asylum..."

"Never!" Amworth retorted. "We can't put her in some filthy madhouse. We must set up a household for her at Warfield. Find a kind widow among the family connections to look after her. In a safe, happy home, she may gradually improve."

Grahame shook his head but didn't argue the point. As an army officer he'd seen madness and knew it came in many forms, including

3

total withdrawal from the real world. He doubted that Lady Meriel Grahame, only child of the fifth Earl Grahame, would ever regain her sanity. But Amworth was right; she could be kept in comfort. It was the least—and the most—her uncles could do.

When news of the small heiress was released, people talked about what a miracle the child's survival was. But such a pity what had happened to her.

Such a pity.

Chapter 1

Dominic Renbourne's head was pounding like a regimental drum. He came awake slowly, knowing he shouldn't have drunk so much at the boxing match the night before. A good evening, but he'd pay for it all day.

Belatedly he realized there was pounding on the door as well as in his head. Where the hell was Clement? Damn, his valet was still in the country visiting his ailing mother. Bloody nuisance.

Since the knocking showed no sign of abatement, Dominic swung his legs to the floor and took stock. The sun's rays said early afternoon, not morning. He still wore crumpled breeches and shirt, but had managed to get his coat and boots off before collapsing on the bed.

Yawning, he ambled from his bedroom into

the sitting room. He hoped Clement's mother recovered soon; Dominic's rooms were a shambles. If matters got much worse, he'd have to find a charwoman to clean the place.

He swung open the door and saw—himself.

Or rather, a cold-eyed, immaculately tailored version of himself. The shock of seeing his twin brother in the passageway was like a splash of ice water.

Before Dominic could think of a suitably acid greeting, his brother pushed past him into the sitting room. "You need a shave and a haircut." Kyle kicked aside a rumpled coat with one shining black boot. "And a bonfire to purge this place."

"I don't recall asking your opinion." Dominic's normally easy temper flared with the special kind of irritation that only his brother and father could inspire. How long had it been since he'd seen Kyle? At least two years, and then only in passing, with cool nods exchanged. They didn't move in the same circles. Both of them preferred it that way. "Why are you here? Has Wrexham died?"

"The earl enjoys his usual health. Robust, in an invalidish sort of way." His brother began to prowl the room, unease showing in every line of his body.

Dominic closed the door, then leaned against it and folded his arms across his chest, beginning to enjoy his twin's obvious discomfort. Kyle had always concealed a tense, restless nature under a rigidly controlled exterior, but today the control was slipping

5

badly. He looked ready to jump out of his skin. "If our dear father is still among the living, why are you stooping to visit my poor chambers?"

Kyle frowned. In another few years his sour disposition would carve hard lines around his mouth, yet for now his features were still eerily like the image Dominic saw in the mirror every morning. Kyle's face was a fraction fuller, his eyes perhaps a shade less blue, but the pair of them were still alike as peas in a pod. Both a little above middle height, leanly built but with broad shoulders, dark hair with a slight wave. As a boy, Dominic had reveled in that resemblance. Now he resented it. It seemed wrong that they should appear so similar when they were utterly different.

"Perhaps I am visiting from brotherly affection."

"Do you think I'm a fool, Lord Maxwell?"

"Yes," his brother said bluntly, his contemptuous gaze scanning the cluttered room. "Surely you can do better than this with your life."

Dominic's mouth hardened. His manner of living was not a subject he would discuss with his brother. "I presume you are here because you want something, though I can't imagine what a useless younger son could possibly offer to the lord and heir of Wrexham." And if Kyle did want something, he was going about it the wrong way.

Apparently realizing that, his brother said in a more moderate tone, "You're right, I need help, and only you can supply it."

6

"Indeed?"

His eyes showing how much he hated asking for aid, Kyle said flatly, "I want you to pretend to be me for several weeks."

After a moment of shock, Dominic laughed. "Don't be absurd. I could fool strangers easily enough, but not anyone who knows you well. Besides, what is the point? Deception is a child's game." Dominic had always been better at impersonating his brother than the other way around, but they hadn't changed places since they'd started school. Or rather, schools. Sometimes Dominic wondered how different his life would have been if they'd both gone to Eton.

"There are...special circumstances. You would be among strangers, not anyone who knows me." Kyle hesitated, then added, "I'll make it worth your while."

Dominic had been heading toward the small butler's pantry, but at that he swung around, eyes glittering. "Out. *Now.*" Though he had been bullied and betrayed by his brother, he would never be bought.

Kyle pulled a folded sheaf of papers from an inside pocket and tossed them at Dominic. "Your reward if you carry this off successfully."

Dominic caught the sheaf and opened it, then stopped in his tracks, stunned by what he held. "This is the deed to Bradshaw Manor!"

"I'm quite aware of what it is." Kyle plucked the deed from his brother's hand and tucked it back inside his coat.

As a younger son, Dominic received a

modest allowance, barely enough to live as a gentleman, while Kyle would eventually receive the entire Wrexham fortune. Quite a reward for emerging from their mother's body a mere ten minutes earlier. And not only would Kyle someday be one of Britain's great lords, on their twenty-first birthday he had received Bradshaw Manor outright. It was a fine estate in Cambridgeshire, well cultivated and including a handsome house. Dominic would sell his soul for Bradshaw Manor— and Kyle knew it. "You *bastard*."

"I could hardly be illegitimate without you being the same, dear brother." Kyle smiled as he saw the power shifting into his hands. "And you malign our mother, of hallowed memory."

Dominic's response was unprintable. Kyle had him, and they both knew it. In dire need of refreshment, he stepped in the pantry and pulled a jug of ale from the cupboard, then poured a full measure into a tankard that was fairly clean. He did not offer his brother a drink.

After a deep swig, Dominic returned to the sitting room, claiming the most comfortable chair. "Explain why you want me to play the role of Lord Maxwell."

His brother began to pace again. "When we were boys, Wrexham and the fifth Earl Grahame talked of a match between me and Grahame's daughter."

Dominic nodded. It was one of the times he'd been grateful to be a younger son. But the plan had been dropped. He thought a moment. "Isn't the girl mad?"

"She's not mad," Kyle said sharply. "Just...different."

It sounded as if his brother had met the girl and liked what he saw. "Do you mean she's merely eccentric? If so, she'd make a fine Renbourne."

Kyle stopped at the window, staring out at soot-stained London chimneys. "Earl Grahame was in India on a political mission when he and his wife were killed by bandits. Lady Meriel was taken captive. She was only five. More than a year passed before she was restored to the British authorities, and by then the damage was done. Her ordeal changed her into a mute lost in some private world, but she is no raving lunatic."

That was far beyond eccentric. "The fact that she doesn't rave doesn't make her sane," Dominic exclaimed. "You're willing to bed a lunatic for her fortune? Jesus, Kyle, that's disgusting."

"It's not like that!" Kyle swung around angrily before recapturing his control. "Though I'll admit that Wrexham favors the match because she's an heiress."

"I always knew he was greedy, but I'm amazed that he's willing to sully the noble Renbourne line with a madwoman's blood."

"He discussed the matter with her physicians. Since she was born a healthy, normal child, there is no reason to suppose that her children will be afflicted."

Dominic's lips curled with distaste. "This all sounds like an elaborate rationalization to disguise the fact that the two of you will do anything for money. Does marriage really mean so little to you, Kyle?"

His brother flushed. "This isn't about money. Lady Meriel will suit me well."

"Where do I come into this pretty picture?" Dominic swallowed a generous mouthful of ale. "Do you need help in bedding your idiot bride? It's true that I'm very good at bedding. You, I suppose, have never stooped to anything so undignified as making the beast with two backs."

"*Damn* you, Dominic!" Kyle's hands knotted into fists. "You badly need a lesson in manners."

"Perhaps, but not from you," Dominic said coolly. "I ask again—what do you want of me?"

His brother took a slow breath, visibly wrestling with his temper. "The betrothal has not yet been announced because her guardian, Lord Amworth, wishes me to spend several weeks at Lady Meriel's estate to become acquainted with her. If the girl shows signs of dislike, the marriage is off, and I presume he'll look for a different groom."

Dominic grinned maliciously. "And you know yourself to be so charmless that you wish me to substitute and win the poor girl's cooperation in this travesty."

"By God, I knew it was a mistake to come to you," Kyle pivoted and stalked toward the door.

Seeing that he'd gone too far, Dominic

raised a hand to stop him. "Sorry. You shouldn't have called when I have an aching head. I'll grant that you need no help with your wooing—girls always fancied you." Heirs to earldoms were always vastly popular, but Dominic didn't point that out. Any more insults, and he'd never learn what was so important it was worth Bradshaw Manor. "Why do you need my help?"

Kyle wavered a moment before expedience won. "I have another...obligation. Since I can't be in two places at once, I want you to go to Warfield."

Dominic stared at him. "Good God, Kyle, what can be more important than becoming better acquainted with the girl you intend to marry? You need to be there yourself, to decide if you truly wish to make such a strange match. How can I possibly substitute for you?"

"My other obligation is none of your concern," his brother snapped. "As to your relationship with Meriel, though it's probably a stretch to assume you're a gentleman, anyone who rescued as many broken-winged birds as you is unlikely to injure an innocent, unless you've changed beyond all recognition."

Dominic clamped his jaw shut on an automatic retort, knowing it was a mistake to let Kyle anger him. Thinking regretfully of Bradshaw Manor, he made the obvious suggestion. "Surely the best solution is to postpone your visit to Warfield until your other business is finished. Or vice versa."

"Neither can be delayed." Kyle's brows drew together, dark and intimidating. It had been so long since the two of them had spent any time together that Dominic found it unnerving to see his own mannerisms reproduced by his brother. Their habits should have diverged more by now.

"Lady Meriel has two guardians, brothers to her mother and father," Kyle explained. "Her maternal uncle, Lord Amworth, is the one who supports the match. He believes that the right husband, and perhaps children, might help her become normal."

"Surely after so many years, that's unlikely."

"I suspect that Amworth's secret wish is for Meriel to have children. He was very close to his sister—this might be his way of trying to get her back, or at least continuing her line."

Dominic repressed a shiver of distaste. "I suppose that makes sense in an unwholesome way, but why the hurry? If you're the selected stud, a few weeks' delay shouldn't make much difference."

"There is a complication. Her paternal uncle, Lord Grahame, is opposed to the idea of Lady Meriel being wed. He considers it a travesty, a sin against nature."

Dominic agreed with that wholeheartedly. "So Amworth wants the deed done before Grahame finds out. It appears that you risk becoming involved in what could become a nasty scandal."

"Lady Meriel is twenty-three. No court has declared her unfit, so technically she doesn't need her guardians' permission to wed." Despite his smooth explanation, Kyle looked uncomfortable as he continued, "Amworth assures me that Grahame will accept a fait accompli as long as the girl seems content with the result. Since Grahame is traveling on the Continent, Amworth wants his niece wedded and bedded before he returns."

"Why do you want this match, Kyle? There are other heiresses, most of whom would provide you with a more acceptable relationship. Surely you can't have fallen in love with a mute madwoman."

His brother's face hardened. "Lady Meriel is my preference. We will both benefit by the marriage, I believe."

It still sounded like a devilish bad bargain to Dominic, but he and his brother saw things very differently. Their own parents had lived largely separate lives, and apparently Kyle wished to do the same. "I still don't see how a substitution could be done successfully. Oh, I could certainly play a convincing Lord Maxwell for people who don't know you, but I can't live at this estate for weeks, then have you step in without the difference being noticed."

"Lady Meriel lives with a pair of vague old cousins and a household of servants. No one who matters. Simply keep to yourself, avoid becoming intimate with anyone, and spend enough time with the girl so that she is comfortable in your presence."

"She most of all is likely to notice a substitution," Dominic said, exasperated. "Even our dogs and horses could tell us apart instantly."

"She...doesn't notice people. I made a brief visit to Warfield." Kyle fell silent for a moment. "At dinner, she glanced at me once and returned to her soup. I doubt she'll see the difference between you and me."

Dominic tried to imagine a wedding night with a girl who behaved like a wax doll. "This sounds more like rape than marriage."

"Damn you, Dom, I didn't come to listen to your objections!" Kyle exploded. "Will you help me, or not?"

The whip-crack words made Dominic recognize what he should have known the minute his brother walked into the room: Kyle was suffering. Under his arrogance something was terribly wrong. A love affair so unhappy that he literally didn't care who he married? Once Dominic could have asked, but his brother would not answer, not the way things stood between them now.

Equally clear was how desperate Kyle was to get Dominic's cooperation. Granted, someday his brother would be an earl and Bradshaw Manor merely a minor holding, but the estate was still a huge payment for a few weeks of work.

Despite the friction between them, Dominic didn't like seeing his twin so upset. As much because of that as for the potent lure of acquiring his own property, he said, "Very well. I'll do as you ask."

Kyle sighed with relief. "Good. I'm expected at Warfield on Monday, so there isn't much time to prepare you."

"So soon?"

"Do you have business so urgent that you can't leave town right away?"

No, blast it, he didn't. He'd have to cry off a couple of dinner engagements, and his friends would miss him in a casual way, but there was nothing and no one to whom his presence was vital.

As a younger son, Dominic had gone into the army just in time to be blooded at Waterloo. Though he hadn't disgraced himself, the experience had taught him he wasn't cut out to be a soldier. Worse, the peacetime army had proved damned boring.

So he'd sold his commission and lived the carefree life of a young gentleman ever since. The heady delights of London during the Season, and long lazy visits to the country homes of friends the rest of the year. He was just reckless enough to be considered dashing, and innately prudent enough not to get himself into serious trouble. But he was twenty-eight now, and beginning to tire of having no purpose beyond pleasure. Of never doing anything that mattered.

If he owned Bradshaw Manor, his life would have meaning. The broad, fertile fields, the spacious stables and gracious house—the yearning was so sharp he could taste it. "I'll be ready. What needs doing?"

"First, a haircut," his brother said dryly. "Plus

you'll have to take some of my clothing. Your tailor leaves much to be desired."

Dominic made a mental note to "accidentally" wreck at least one of his brother's overpriced coats before this escapade was over. "Anything else?"

"Morrison will go with you. He'll be the only one who knows of the substitution."

Dominic almost groaned aloud. Morrison was as stuffy a valet as Kyle was a master. "Can Morrison get in touch with you if necessary?"

Kyle hesitated. "He'll know where I am, but it will be almost impossible to reach me. I will probably be gone three to five weeks. I expect you to cover for my absence in whatever way is necessary. When you've built an adequate relationship with Lady Meriel, leave. The less time you spend at Warfield, the less likely anyone is to notice the differences between us."

That Dominic agreed with heartily. "Clothing, haircut, valet. I'll also need to know about your meetings with Amworth and your visit to Warfield."

"A good point. I'll make notes." Kyle frowned. "You can't come to Wrexham House—the servants would be shocked to see us on visiting terms. Morrison and I will return tonight with clothing and the information you need. He'll cut your hair then."

Dominic repressed a sigh. It took so little for his brother's natural high-handedness to bloom. "One thing. I want a signed letter from you saying that Bradshaw Manor is mine if I accomplish the goal we have discussed."

Kyle had been about to leave, but at that he swung around, his eyes dangerous. "You doubt my word, Dominic?"

Oddly enough, he did not. "No, but if you get thrown by a horse and killed on this mysterious mission, I'd like to get my payment."

Kyle's brows rose sardonically. "If that happens, brother dear, you're the next Earl of Wrexham, and I wish you much joy of your inheritance."

Then he stalked out the door, closing it hard behind him.

Chapter 2

She entered her workroom from the garden, a bucketful of wildflowers in her left hand. After setting the bucket on the pine table, she contemplated the shelf above, which contained an odd assortment of containers. The cylindrical pottery jar? No, the tall silver coffee pot that she'd taken from the cabinet in the dining room.

Begin with branches of honeysuckle, spiky and heavy with scent.

The door to the conservatory opened behind her and a small, pleasantly plump woman with pure white hair entered. "There's news, dear," Mrs. Rector said in her gentle voice. "Remember that nice young man who came to dinner and spent the night about a fortnight ago? Dark hair, and such a distinguished air? Lord Maxwell."

What to go with the honeysuckle? Masses of speedwell with tiny, vivid blue blossoms. She pulled a handful from the bucket and trimmed the stems with her shears. The curving silver surface of the coffee pot reflected the colors in rich, strange distortions.

Mrs. Rector continued, "Long ago, Lord Maxwell's father and your father planned for the two of you to marry, and your uncle Amworth thinks it a good idea. Remember how your uncle mentioned that to you after Maxwell left?" She sighed. "No, of course you don't remember."

Yellow and blue always looked their best together, so she'd picked dandelions. They contrasted strongly with the speedwell, sparking both to vibrant life.

"Lord Maxwell is coming to stay for several weeks, to further his acquaintance with you." Mrs. Rector studied the worktable. "Oh, dear, the Germain coffee pot. Of course, you own it, so I suppose if you want to stick in weeds, you can."

Something lacy was needed to moderate between the honeysuckle branches and the flowers. Fennel would be best, but it was too early for fennel, so she would have to make do with stitchwort. She slid the gangly stems carefully into the pot, rearranging them until they pleased her.

"As I was saying, Lord Maxwell will arrive on Monday. Your uncle has promised me that the marriage will not take place unless you are comfortable with his lordship."

She turned the pot on the bench, careful to avoid smudging the bright silver with her fingers. Move this bit of honeysuckle *so*. A slight rearrangement of the dandelions, more speedwell *there*.

"I don't see how any good can come of this!" Mrs. Rector burst out. "An innocent like you to wed a worldly man like Lord Maxwell. I swear, I've seen icicles warmer than that man's eyes."

Meriel picked up the arrangement, regarded the effect for a moment, then turned on her stool and placed the coffee pot in Mrs. Rector's hands. The older woman blinked, startled, then smiled. "Why, thank you, my dear. That's so kind of you. It really is rather pretty, isn't it? I shall put it on the dinner table."

She brushed a light kiss on top of Meriel's head. "I shan't let that man hurt you, Meriel, I swear it!" she said in a voice suddenly intense. "I will send a message to Lord Grahame if necessary."

Meriel stood and reached up for the cylindrical pottery jar. The surface was rough, in shades of brown and bronze. It needed lots of dandelions, and yarrow.

Her momentary fierceness gone, Mrs. Rector said uncertainly, "But perhaps Lord Amworth is right. A husband might be just the thing for you. And perhaps a baby." Longing sounded in her voice.

More dandelions were needed. Without a

backward glance at her companion, she slid from the stool and went outside to pick them.

Kyle let himself into the small, elegant town house with his own key. The physician, gray haired and tired eyed, was just leaving. He inclined his head. "My lord."

"Sir George." Kyle set his hat on a side table, which allowed him to hide his expression. "How is she?"

The older man shrugged. "Resting. The laudanum helps with the pain."

In other words, nothing had changed. Not that Kyle expected any miracles. "How long does she have?"

The physician hesitated. "That's always hard to say, but if I had to guess, I'd say perhaps a fortnight."

God willing, that would be long enough. He hoped so with every fiber of his being. "May I see her now?"

"She's awake, though weak. Try not to tire her." The doctor sighed. "Though I suppose it doesn't really matter. Good day, my lord."

After the physician left, Kyle went upstairs, the carpeted steps quiet beneath his feet. How many times had he climbed this staircase? Beyond counting. The moment he first stepped into the little jewel box of a house, he'd known it was perfect for her. She had pronounced herself enchanted, saying that she never wanted to leave. And she hadn't, until these last painful months, when her thoughts had turned elsewhere.

He tapped on the door to warn her before entering. Constancia reclined in a nest of pillows on the sofa, sunshine pouring over her. The harsh light cruelly revealed her ravaged face and the white streaks in her black hair, yet her smile held all the world's sweetness. "Milord. It is good to see you," she said in her seductively accented voice.

He kissed her forehead, then sat in the chair by the sofa and took her hand. It felt unbearably fragile, scarcely more than skin and bones. "I've a surprise for you, Constancia. I've hired a fast private yacht. On Monday, we will sail for Spain on the tide. You'll stay in the captain's own cabin."

She gasped. "How is this possible? You have so many responsibilities. The trip to Shropshire that cannot be delayed..."

"That will be taken care of by my brother."

"Your brother?" Her eyes rounded. "I did not know you had a brother."

For years Kyle had deliberately refrained from mentioning his brother, but that was no longer possible. "Dominic. My twin."

"*Un hermano gemelo?* A twin brother?" she repeated, amazed and intrigued, as people too often were by twins. "Does he look like you?"

"We were considered identical."

She laughed a little. "Two such handsome men! The mind cannot grasp it."

Perhaps that was why he had never mentioned Dominic, his easy-tempered twin, the one who was well liked, especially by women.

21

"Only our faces are alike. In other ways, we are very dissimilar."

Her levity faded, and she gazed at him with the dark eyes that could see right into his soul. "You have told me of your father, your small sister, your mother of blessed memory, but never of your twin. Why not?"

"He's not part of my life. We never see each other." Discomfited by her unswerving gaze, he added, "Dominic was always rebellious. Irresponsible."

"And yet now, he helps you."

"I'm making it worth his while," Kyle said dryly.

She caught her breath. "Is he pretending to be you? Surely not, *querido!*"

He swore to himself. He hadn't meant her to know this much, but it was hard to keep anything from her quick, intuitive mind. Not wanting to discuss his brother any more, he said, "I'll tell Teresa to start packing your things. There isn't much time."

She closed her eyes for a moment, a shadow of pain crossing her face. "No," she whispered. "Hardly any time left at all."

It wasn't easy to keep his voice steady. "Time enough to take you home, as I promised I would."

"Yes, but I did not think you were serious. For a young lord to lower himself to escorting his old mistress...unthinkable!" With her free hand, she wiped away tears. "*Diablo!* I cry too easily now. How can I take so much from you, *mi corazón,* my heart?"

She had never understood how much he owed her. Constancia de las Torres had been only a girl when she was driven from her home by war, and ravished into the bargain. She had survived in the only way open to a lovely young woman who was destitute and alone. Later, during the Peninsular War, she had accompanied a British officer back to England as his mistress. When the affair ended, she'd become a London courtesan, known publicly as La Paloma. The dove.

She'd been more than twice Kyle's age when he went to her as an eighteen-year-old virgin. He was captivated the first time he saw her in a box at the opera, and not only because of her dark, exotic beauty. Demanding an introduction from a mutual friend, he'd immediately invited her to join him for a late supper after the performance.

Though he tried to act worldly, he couldn't have fooled her for a minute. But Constancia had kept any amusement to herself, welcoming him into her arms with a generosity that made him feel like a man among men.

Even that first time, he'd known that what he had discovered with La Paloma went far beyond the intoxicating pleasures of passion. In a profession that turned most women hard and cold, she had a rare and precious warmth. With her he found peace, and a filling of the emptiness that had been part of him since he and Dominic became estranged. Only much later did he realize that he gave much to her as well. Even so, she'd resisted when he asked her to become his mistress, saying that she was past her prime and a beautiful man like him deserved an equally beautiful young girl.

It was true that she was no longer young, and that she faced a future of increasing bleakness in a trade where youth and beauty were the only coin that mattered. But his desire to keep her safe had been only a small part of his decision; far more important was his fierce need to keep her close, for he could not imagine life without her.

"I've always wanted to go to Spain. You've given me a reason," he said in a light voice that showed none of his thoughts. "We shall lie beneath an orange tree and smell the flowers on the warm Spanish wind."

"Yes." Despite the fatigue in her dark eyes, she gave him her wonderful Madonna smile again. "Surely God will grant me that much."

He smiled back, and wondered with despair what he would ever do without her.

*T*he small boy emerged from his father's study, so stunned that he knew only that control was essential. Shoulders rigid, he walked through the grand hall, steps echoing, then down the wide stone steps after a footman silently swung the door open.

Kyle raced around the corner, face alive with excitement. "Did you fool him?"

Dominic licked his dry lips. "Oh, yes, he thought I was you."

His brother grinned mischievously. "I told you

24

Wrexham couldn't tell us apart, even though he is our father."

Dominic could no longer remember why the idea of trying to deceive the earl had seemed amusing. "Of course he can't. He hardly ever sees us, and he's shortsighted as an owl."

Catching his mood, Kyle frowned. "What's wrong? Was I summoned for punishment and you got beaten in my place? Honest, Dom, I wouldn't have suggested tricking him if I thought that's what he was going to do!"

"Not a beating. Worse." Dominic glanced at the broad, grimly impressive facade of Dornleigh, chilled to the heart. "Race you to the gazebo. I'll tell you there."

He took off running, his twin a half step behind. By the time they reached the circular Greek temple that presided over the gardens, both were panting with effort. Fiercely competitive, Kyle dived the last few feet, his hand slapping the bottom stone step just as Dominic reached it. "I'm first!"

"No, you're not!" Chest heaving, Dominic glared at his brother, but his protest was halfhearted. He turned and dropped onto the top step, his blind gaze not seeing the lush greenery. "He...he's going to send us to different schools."

"What!" Kyle sank onto the step beside him. "He can't do that!"

"He can, and has." Dominic swallowed, afraid tears might start. "Come Michaelmas, you're going to Eton, while I'm being packed off to Rugby."

He felt the silent wave of pain from his brother, an echo of his own horror when Wrexham had made the announcement. His earliest memories were of

Kyle. He could sooner imagine cutting off his right arm than living apart from his twin. "Maybe Mama can change his mind."

"He never listens to her," Kyle retorted. "He never listens to anybody."

Too true to be argued. "I'll get myself sent down from Rugby. Then maybe he'll let me go to Eton, too."

"He'll beat you, but he won't send you to Eton." Kyle frowned. "In a way, it makes sense. After all, I'm going to be the earl, and the Earls of Wrexham have always gone to Eton." His assessing gaze scanned the Northamptonshire hills, Wrexham land as far as the eye could see. "You're only a younger son."

"Just because you're ten minutes older!" Dominic's distress turned into rage, and he launched himself at his brother, fists flying.

"I'm the heir and you're the spare!" Kyle taunted, striking back. "It was me he called in to discuss our schooling. You were only there because we tricked him."

The two of them rolled across the grass, kicking and hitting in one of the swift, violent conflicts that sometimes flared up between them. The fight ended when a shove sent Kyle's head against a stone step, and he went limp.

Panicked, Dominic dropped to his knees beside his brother. Blood was flowing from a gash above Kyle's ear. Dominic yanked out a handkerchief and pressed the folded fabric to the bloodstained dark hair. "Kyle, are you all right?"

His twin blinked dazedly. "I'm still ten minutes older than you, Dom."

Dominic sank back on his heels, relieved. Holding the pad to the gash, he said, "Older isn't better."

"Ten minutes better, but because of that, I get beaten more often." A glimmer of smile faded swiftly. "Maybe we should run away."

It was Dominic's turn to be reasonable. "He can send us to different schools, but he can't separate us, not really. We're two halves of the same whole."

Kyle gave Dominic a fierce one-armed hug. "And best friends. Always."

At the age of ten, neither of them could imagine an end to their closeness.

Dominic came awake, heart pounding. It had been years since he'd dreamed of that day when everything changed. Kyle's sudden reappearance in his life had triggered the memories again. That summer before they started school had been the last good time before life went wrong.

Not wrong, he reminded himself forcefully. That had been the beginning of his freedom to be himself, rather than a useless appendage of the Renbourne family. Despite Kyle's wealth and great expectations, Dominic wouldn't want to change places, not really. Living under Wrexham's thumb was enough to make anyone bad-tempered. Bad-tempered, and damned arrogant.

Now Dominic would have to imitate that stiffness. Wonderful. With a sigh, he got up from the bed. Dawn was showing in the east, and soon Morrison would arrive with Kyle's carriage for the trip to Shropshire, north and west by the Welsh border. A trunk was packed with Kyle's clothing, though not his boots. Dominic's feet, like his face, were a fraction narrower, so he preferred his own footwear.

He washed and shaved himself—did Kyle know how to shave, or did the estimable Morrison always do it for him?—then dressed. He was just finishing a hasty breakfast of bread, cheese, and ale when his brother's valet arrived.

Slight of build and of indeterminate age, Morrison said, "I trust you are ready for departure, my lord."

He had the schoolmaster's trick of making every remark sound vaguely censorious. A good thing Kyle's favorite horse was tethered behind the carriage, so Dominic could ride when the mood struck him.

Using Kyle's clipped inflections, he replied, "Quite ready, Morrison."

The valet blinked, startled, as Dominic caught up his brother's dark cloak and led the way into the common passageway that served four floors' worth of "rooms for gentlemen." As he locked his door behind him, he was struck by the sense that he was locking away the Honorable Dominic Renbourne. From this moment, he was Lord Maxwell, arrogant viscount, a man utterly sure of his place in the world.

The thought was surprisingly upsetting. He had a sudden crazy desire to say, "Sorry,

I've changed my mind. Kyle will have to court his own bride." After which he'd toss the cloak over Morrison's disapproving face and go back into his rooms. They might be cluttered, but they were *his*.

But if there was one thing the Renbourne sons had in common, it was that they were both men of their word. Dominic became very still, consciously making the subtle adjustments that would produce Kyle's harder step and less expressive face. It wasn't enough to use his brother's voice; he must learn to think his brother's thoughts.

Then, when he had become Lord Maxwell, he went down the steps ready to deceive.

Chapter 3

Late May was full of promises, the richest, most fertile time of the year. All nature was in bloom and wild beasts ecstatically sought their mates. Meriel had discarded her slippers in favor of living earth beneath her toes. Since early morning she'd been working in the herb garden, pruning and dividing to keep the plants healthy.

Some of the herbs were ancient, planted by long-forgotten ancestors. The marjoram had surely been placed in this spot by a woman who tended her herbs just as Meriel did now, raising potent plants for healing and cooking. When Meriel was small, Kamal had studied an old herbal in the library, then described the plants and their uses to her when they worked here. He'd been a wonderful teacher, his deep, slow voice making all subjects interesting as he spoke. His manner had been casual, as if he were talking to himself. Did he know how much she had learned that way? Impossible to say.

She finished in the herb garden by midafternoon. The day being ripe with scent and sun, she snapped her fingers for her dog, Roxana, who lay dozing by the rosemary. Together they strolled through the park toward Warfield's main entrance. She loved the diamond-shaped gatehouse towers, and the arch that leaped between them above the road. The gateway was built of the same warm gray stone as the wall that circled the park, enclosing her world in a circle of safety.

Within sight of the gateway, she found a favorite hidden spot between two rhododendron bushes on the verge of coming into bloom. She settled down on crossed legs, Roxana flopping beside her, and lazily studied the elaborately whorled wrought iron gates that filled the arch. The iron was painted a glossy black, except for several spikes at the top that glittered with gold leaf. Sometimes she wondered about the land of Others that lay beyond the gates, though not with any desire to visit. Too much of what she remembered was horror. Pain and glare and fire in the night.

Dreamily her mind drifted, absorbing the

essence of the day. Light wind trembled the ivy that twined up the towers and along the wall, while thrushes sang in the nearby trees. How would it feel to be a rhododendron, sinking roots into the rich, dark soil, drawing life from the sun and the rain? Or a thrush, darting through the air... ? She slid into the golden place at the center of her being where all nature was one.

Shadows were lengthening when her attention was brought back by a horseman cantering up to the gates. Neatly he pulled his horse around and tugged at the bell rope. Intrigued, she waited without impatience to see what would happen.

More restless, horse and rider paced in rough circles until old Walter, the gatekeeper, emerged from his sitting room in the right-hand gate tower. As soon as he saw the visitor, he bobbed his head, then opened the gates.

Meriel felt a sudden chill when she saw the man more clearly. He had come once before, not long ago. His gaze had been sharp as cut glass, but he'd left quickly. A man of no importance.

Now he had returned, and there was something different about him. He no longer seemed like someone who could be easily ignored.

Roxana whimpered. Meriel stilled the dog with one hand, eyes narrowed as she studied the newcomer. Hatless, wind-blown hair waving across a sweaty brow, a suggestion of cleft in his chin. What would be considered a handsome face. His bay horse was equally splendid, a brown dark almost to black. A shade very like the rider's hair, in fact. Both were magnificent beasts.

He exchanged a few words with the gatekeeper, then turned his mount and scanned his surroundings. Instinctively she shrank back as his gaze went over her hiding place. His eyes were intensely blue, like cornflowers, visible even at this distance. She held her breath until he started up the drive. Man and horse moved in perfect harmony, smooth muscles working under glossy hide, the rider effortlessly controlling the powerful animal between his legs.

She drew up her knees and locked her arms around them, rocking back and forth in disquiet. Most of the males who worked at Warfield were middle-aged or older, but this one was young and virile, in the prime of life. A man used to getting his way by natural right. One who rode like a conqueror.

He must have come to dine with the ladies again. She'd not go to the meal. At this season, there was scarcely any reason to enter the house at all. She could sleep in the tree house and forage for food.

Yes, she'd stay away until the man left, for her home would not be the same while he was here.

The long drive from London had been a bore, but Kyle's horse, Pegasus, was a treat. With Warfield near, Dominic saddled the beast and rode ahead, reaching his destination well

32

before the dour Morrison and the lumbering coach. The gatekeeper remembered him—or rather, Kyle—and greeted him with frank interest. The story of Lady Meriel's betrothal must be known to the servants.

He trotted leisurely to the house along an avenue shaded by great spreading lime trees. The park, the semicultivated area surrounding the house, was a magnificent expanse of rolling landscape. Trees and shrubs were scattered across the velvety green turf, while grazing cows and small, shy deer kept the grass trim and the trees free of branches up to the height of a cow's head.

Except for a section bounded by the river, this particular park was entirely walled in, according to Kyle. Convenient for keeping mad girls from wandering off.

Dominic reined in Pegasus when the house came into sight. Built of the same gray stone as the park wall, it was a sprawling, symmetrical structure with gables and a steep-pitched slate roof. A hundred and fifty years or so old, he guessed.

The formal seat of the Earls Grahame was in Lincolnshire, on the other side of England. Meriel's uncle lived there, but her parents had preferred Warfield, which had been in the family of Meriel's mother for centuries. Presumably Kyle would let his wife stay here in her familiar home after they married, while he himself spent most of his time at Dornleigh or in London. He could visit when he felt the need for a child or two.

Mouth tight, Dominic guided Pegasus around the house to the stables. No one was in sight. He dismounted and led the horse inside. Though the building was large, only a handful of stalls were occupied, mostly by aging carriage horses.

He glanced around, wondering if he'd have to rub down his own horse. He wouldn't mind; in fact, he preferred caring for his beasts himself, but Kyle would expect better service. Then a groom as elderly as the gatekeeper creaked into view. "G'day, Lord Maxwell." He bobbed his head respectfully. "Shall I take your horse?"

Dominic passed over his reins. He almost added a casual comment about the fine weather, then bit the words back. Kyle was not given to conversation with unknown servants. It also belatedly occurred to him that his brother would not have left his hat in the carriage, as Dominic had.

After explaining that his luggage would arrive later, he made his way toward the house, reviewing what he'd been told about the household, for this was the most critical stage of his visit. Lady Meriel was supervised by two elderly widows, distant cousins of some sort. Mrs. Rector and Mrs. Marks. Kyle had been dismissive of the pair, saying they would be easily deceived.

Dominic was less sure. In his experience, little old ladies were often observant, especially since Kyle's visit would have been an exciting event in an otherwise quiet life.

As he reached the bottom of the steps, the door opened and two women emerged, smiling in welcome. The smaller one was soft and round and sweetly fey, with very white hair. The other was taller, with an angular face and hair blended of brown and silvery gray. He realized with alarm that he hadn't the vaguest idea which was which.

The angular woman said, "Lord Maxwell, so good to see you again. I trust your journey was pleasant."

Uneasily he recognized that the shrewd hazel eyes behind her spectacles wouldn't miss much. Damnation, which cousin was she?

Reminding himself to be as cool as Kyle, he bowed deeply. "As you can see, I couldn't resist riding ahead. My man will be along soon with my carriage."

The other woman said solicitously, "You must be tired. Would you like a nice cup of tea?"

"It would be my pleasure." He took both ladies' arms, making them smile, and escorted them up the steps. "Will Lady Meriel be joining us?"

"Oh, no," the taller one said, sounding as if the answer was so obvious that the question shouldn't be asked. Despite his preparation, Dominic was alarmingly aware of how much he didn't know. This place, these women, were strangers.

And he should have worn the damned hat.

The arrival of Morrison and the baggage allowed Dominic to put himself into a more Kyle-ish frame of mind for dinner. He dressed with careful formality, as befitted a man about to meet his bride, then studied himself in the mirror. Remarkable how different tailoring and subtle changes in expression altered that image. Only someone who knew Kyle well would realize that the mirror reflected a different man.

A dinner bell rang with a clamor to wake the dead, so he descended to the small salon, where his two hostesses awaited. He'd hoped to meet his brother's betrothed as well, but she wasn't there. After sherry and a brief exchange of pleasantries, he escorted the ladies in to dinner. Four places were set. Still no Lady Meriel. The angular woman—he'd forgotten to ask Morrison to identify the ladies—frowned at the empty chair, then signaled for the meal to begin.

Apart from an odd centerpiece composed of weeds, the meal and service were excellent, but the fourth chair remained obstinately empty. Dominic knew that Kyle's one brief meeting with his intended bride had been at this dinner table, so finally he asked, "Is Lady Meriel unwell?"

The two women exchanged glances again. The smaller one said uncomfortably, "You know how she is, Lord Maxwell. Usually she dines with us, but not always."

He took a sip of wine as he thought. Deciding on frankness even though it was more his

36

style than his brother's, he said, "But I don't really know how she is. Though I've met the girl and discussed her with Lord Amworth, that's not the same as personal knowledge. Perhaps this would be a good time for you to tell me more about her. After all, you two know her best."

"I suppose you're right, though no one really knows her, except perhaps Kamal." The smaller woman turned her earnest gaze on him. "Meriel is not like anyone else. She's such a sweet child."

"Not a child," her companion corrected. "A woman grown. That's one reason Amworth wishes to see her wed—he fears that in her innocence, she might be led astray."

Dominic absorbed that. "Are you saying that she has no moral sense?"

"How can she?" It was the angular woman again. "She has the mind of a child. No, not even that, for even an infant will respond to human contact. Meriel—" she hesitated, groping for words—"she scarcely sees us at all. She's like a sweet-tempered ghost who lives in her own world, separate from the rest of mankind."

"Except when she has a tantrum," the smaller woman said tartly. "I shall be frank with you, my lord. I have doubts about the wisdom of this match. I don't think that Meriel can even understand the concept of marriage, nor can I imagine how you would find such a union satisfactory by any standard."

He studied the soft round face and faded blue

eyes, and decided that anyone who thought little old ladies were negligible wasn't paying attention. "I appreciate your frankness. Remember, the match has not yet taken place. The purpose of this visit is to confirm that marriage is feasible. I assure you that I mean the girl no harm."

The small woman nodded, satisfied, but Dominic was troubled. Kyle had seemed determined to make this marriage. Though Dominic shouldn't care what stupidity his brother committed, he did care, blast it. He was going to have to try to ingratiate himself with the girl while leaving the situation open enough to allow Kyle to withdraw honorably if he changed his mind. "What is the range of Lady Meriel's abilities?"

"She has a gift for working with plants and animals." The taller woman smiled sadly. "Perhaps that is because she is closer to the beasts of the field than she is to humankind. Heaven knows she completely lacks normal understanding. Look at these flowers." She indicated the arrangement of dandelions and other weeds that sat in the middle of the polished mahogany table in a crude ceramic jug. "Meriel made this. It is a more eloquent statement of her personality than any description Ada or I can make."

Progress; he would ask Morrison which of the ladies had Ada for a Christian name. But he understood the woman's point when he gazed at the centerpiece. Most women of gentle birth prided themselves on being able to create attractive floral arrangements for their homes. Even the coarsest village girl could brighten a cottage with flowers from her garden. This bouquet was pathetic. Not only was it composed of common weeds, but the wildflowers she'd chosen had such a short life that by tomorrow they would be dead, and all her efforts wasted after only a few hours.

He felt a sharp pang of regret for the bright child whose mind had been destroyed by a horror that sealed her tongue forever. If her family had not died in a savage attack, Lady Meriel would probably be married now, perhaps a mother. Instead, even her guardians considered her scarcely more than a wild beast.

The thought of spending time with this warped travesty of humanity was deeply unappealing, but he was here to lie for his brother, so he said gallantly, "I look forward to furthering my acquaintance with Lady Meriel. Perhaps a new influence in her life will bring about improvement."

From the ladies' expressions, they didn't believe that any more than he did.

Chapter 4

After dressing the next morning, Dominic lingered at the window of his spacious bedchamber. He was placed at the back of the house, and from this height he could look over Warfield's vast gardens. Varied like a patchwork quilt, they extended for many acres. Directly behind the house was a parterre, a formal garden of clipped hedges and flower beds divided by mellow brick paths. The over-all design was a Maltese cross centered on a splendid multitiered fountain.

Morrison appeared silently beside him. The man crept about like a rodent.

Dominic turned from the window. "The two ladies—which is which? The smaller one's first name is Ada, but is she Mrs. Marks or Mrs. Rector?"

"She is Mrs. Rector, my lord. The taller female is Mrs. Edith Marks." Morrison cleared his throat with the sound that meant he wished to speak. "When I breakfasted in the servant's hall, I learned that Lady Meriel did not sleep in her room last night."

Dominic frowned. "Were the servants concerned?"

"Not at all. I received the impression that the young lady often sleeps outdoors, especially during mild weather." Disapproval sounded in the valet's voice.

"So she's not even housebroken." Dominic looked Morrison directly in the eye. "What do you think of this proposed marriage?"

The valet's expression became even stiffer than usual. "It is not my place to question my master's personal affairs."

"I'm sure you have opinions, especially about a matter which concerns you so closely," Dominic said, voice edged. "I would appreciate an honest answer."

"I have grave doubts about the wisdom of this, my lord," Morrison said slowly. "Marriage is a lifelong commitment. It should not be undertaken lightly."

The man had more sense than Kyle. "Perhaps your master will reconsider in the next weeks."

Morrison's gaze moved so that he was staring blankly out the window. "If the girl takes a dislike to you, there would be no marriage."

Was the valet suggesting that Dominic deliberately alienate Lady Meriel? Apparently. "I cannot make so important a decision for my brother."

Morrison's gaze dropped, possibly with a hint of disappointment.

The breakfast bell rang. Warfield was a great house for bells. As Dominic went downstairs, he wondered if the ringing was done to summon Lady Meriel for meals. He'd noticed that the bell rang outside as well as in the house.

Of course, summoning her didn't mean that she'd come. The two widows were already seated in the breakfast room, so Dominic greeted them, then helped himself to the dishes on the sideboard. As he piled thinly sliced ham on his plate, he said, "It appears that Lady Meriel has taken me in dislike. Or is she always absent for so long?"

"She does seem to be avoiding you," Mrs. Rector said apologetically. "She is often shy of strangers."

That was an understatement. "Might she stay in hiding until I leave?"

Mrs. Marks said with reluctance, "That could happen."

"Perhaps I should organize a hunt with beaters to drive her into the open like a pheasant," he said dryly as he seated himself at the table.

"Absolutely not." Mrs. Rector's head shot up, a fierceness in her eyes that was at odds with her gentle features. "Oh. I see that you're joking."

Yes, but if he had to wait days for an elusive madwoman to appear, a hunt would start seeming like a good idea. "Do you have any suggestions for how I might find her?"

Mrs. Marks thought about it. "She spends almost all her time in the gardens, though they are so large she could avoid you for days. Warfield has always been famous for its gardens. Every generation has added to them. To find Meriel, you might try watching the tree house. I believe she sleeps there when she isn't in the house."

"Ask Kamal," Mrs. Rector suggested. "He would have the best idea of where to find her. Look for him in the garden sheds after breakfast."

Kyle had mentioned an Indian servant. "Kamal is a gardener?"

Mrs. Rector nodded. "He supervises everything to do with the gardens, because he is the only one who understands what Meriel wants."

Dominic's brows arched. "So she has opinions about her plants?"

"Oh, yes. When she was small, she would have

tantrums if the old head gardener did things she didn't like." She cut a neat piece of coddled egg. "Eventually we let him go and put Kamal in his place. Besides supervising the garden staff, he is our liaison to Mr. Kerr, the steward who runs the home farm and supervises the tenants. I don't know what we should do without Kamal."

Dominic frowned at the mention of tantrums, but there was a positive aspect to what Mrs. Rector had said. "If Lady Meriel has preferences for her garden, she can't be entirely mindless."

"Even a dog will get angry if its routine is changed," Mrs. Marks pointed out. "Her preferences are often...very strange. More proof of her madness, I fear." Her gaze went to the wilting centerpiece, which looked even more grotesque this morning.

Each new piece of information made Lady Meriel sound more hopeless. Repressing a sigh, Dominic got directions to the garden sheds and set out to find them after breakfast. A door at the back of the house opened onto a broad stone patio with steps descending to the parterre he had seen from above. To his left, a large, glassed-in conservatory was attached to the back of the house.

Making a note to investigate the conservatory later, he strolled through the parterre. A pair of peafowl were drinking from the fountain in the center. The cock gave Dominic a beady-eyed stare, then spread his shimmering tail in a way that said, "Top *this*." The hen contented herself with an earsplitting screech.

43

With a smile, Dominic went around them. He'd always liked peafowl. As a boy, he'd bought a pair from a neighbor and proudly given them to his father for Dornleigh. The earl had hated the noise, though. Dominic had enlisted Kyle to help capture the pair and return them to the neighbor before Wrexham ordered the elegant necks wrung.

Following Mrs. Rector's direction, he walked a corner path into a more informal area. Towering walls of smooth clipped yew provided a dark green background for lush borders of blossoming shrubs and flowers. From the varied selection, he guessed that there would be blooming from early spring to first frost.

A wrong turn landed him in a rose garden. He'd never seen so many varieties of roses. The scent was intoxicating.

By the time he reached the gardening sheds, it was midmorning and he'd seen at least four different gardeners at work. Such extensive gardens required endless effort.

He peered into the first shed, which was used for tool storage. No one. The next shed contained bins of various substances to be worked into soil to create different conditions. It was also empty.

Next in the row was a long glasshouse, used to protect tender plants in winter and grow fruits and vegetables year round. Dominic was struck by the heat when he entered, for the glass panels trapped and magnified the effects of the sun. At the far end of the structure, he saw the back of a man standing at a broad workbench, though details were obscured by hanging plants that would do credit to a Brazilian jungle.

As he approached the gardener, he saw that the man wore a turban and a loose, sashed blue cotton tunic that fell over baggy cotton trousers. The Indian garb must be very practical for garden work. "Kamal? I'm Maxwell."

The Indian turned from his repotting. Kamal was broad and strong and fearsomely bearded, and the turban gave him towering height. He was a formidable protector for his mad mistress.

But what startled Dominic most were elaborate tattoos that covered Kamal's hands and forearms with swirls and decorative patterns. Good God, there were even zigzag designs on his throat and on his cheeks above the bushy black whiskers.

"Lord Maxwell." The Indian placed both hands together in front of his chest and inclined his head. *"Namaste."* The gesture was polite, but certainly not deferential.

Dominic said, "Good day. I'm looking for Lady Meriel. Do you have an idea where she might be found?"

The Indian studied him with dark, piercing eyes, weighing his worth. Kyle would have been furious at such a blatant appraisal. Even Dominic felt his hackles rise. "I presume you know why I am here."

"I know, my lord." Kamal said in faintly accented but very fluent English. "You wish to marry the young mistress."

"I seek to discover if marriage is feasible," Dominic said sharply. "That can't be done if I can't find the lady."

"She was in the herb garden." Kamal gestured with his chin. "That way, along the path behind the glass house. But I am not sure. She may have left."

"If she has, I shall return for another suggestion." Dominic left the glass house, glad to get into cooler air.

The path Kamal had indicated was again walled with hedges higher than a man's head, though these were not clipped to unnatural smoothness. The walkway soon opened up into a pleasant herb garden, but the girl wasn't there. Dominic wandered the neat brick paths, noting signs of recent work. Had she seen him coming and fled, or left because she'd finished her task? He bent and pinched a downy leaf from an irregularly shaped blue-gray shrub, releasing a pungent odor. Some kind of mint, he thought.

"Meo-o-o-ow!"

An enormous orange marmalade cat slid sinuously from under a nearby bush. Golden eyes hot with interest, the cat reared up against Dominic's leg and raspily slurped the fingers that had pinched the leaf.

"So this is catmint." Dominic ruffled the orange striped fur. "A good thing you decided to lick, not bite. A tom your size could do serious damage. Would you like some catmint of your own?"

"Meo-o-o-ow." The cat butted his hand.

Taking that as a yes, Dominic went down on one knee and pinched off half a dozen leaves, then crushed them into an aromatic ball and tossed it past the cat. The tom leaped on the catmint with a hunting cry, somersaulting over the path as he shredded the leaves with wicked claws. Then he slashed at the catmint plant itself, demonstrating why the shape was so irregular.

Dominic was about to rise when he glanced up and saw a young woman enter the far end of the garden. Lady Meriel had returned, perhaps drawn by the yowling cat.

He caught his breath, stunned. Gods above, why had no one told him she was beautiful? Petite and graceful, with features as delicately molded as a porcelain doll, Lady Meriel seemed to have stepped from a Renaissance painting, or perhaps the land of Faerie. Ivory-pale hair was pulled back into a wrist-thick braid, and her gaze seemed fixed on visions invisible to the normal run of humankind.

Then she saw him. Her eyes widened with shock before she whirled and bolted from the herb garden like a deer, bare feet flying as she darted back through the opening in the hedge through which she'd come.

"Wait!" He scrambled to his feet and raced after her, but by the time he reached the hedge she'd vanished into an area carefully designed to imitate wilderness. The brick path changed to shredded bark and split into three forks in front of him. He was about to choose one when he realized that pursuit was a damned poor idea if he wanted to win the trust of a shy, wary girl.

Shaken, he returned to the herb garden and sank onto a stone bench set against the encircling hedge. His pulse was pounding, and not from sprinting a few yards. Now that he'd seen her, he understood why Kyle was willing to overlook Lady Meriel's mental state. Merciful heaven, but she was lovely, with a fey, ethereal beauty that could entrance any man. He'd seen hair of such fairness only once before, on an exquisite Norwegian courtesan whose price had been well beyond his purse.

He tried to reconstruct her image from that fleeting glimpse. What color were her eyes? Light, but dark enough to add definition to that small, perfect face. She wore a simple blue tunic over a full skirt in a darker shade of blue. A sash was tied around her waist, rather like Kamal's sash. Was her garb Indian? Perhaps, or it could have been modeled on medieval peasant clothing. The costume gave her an otherworldly quality, as if she belonged to no particular time or place.

As his breathing steadied, he asked himself why beauty made so much difference. Lady Meriel Grahame's sad past and stunted life would be equally tragic if she were ugly as a hedgehog, yet the fact that she was beautiful deepened his regret almost unbearably. Wryly he acknowledged that he must be very shallow. Even knowing that, he could not stop himself from being moved by the memory of her fair, haunting face.

The cure for mystery was familiarity, becoming accustomed to her striking appearance. But how could he manage that when she fled at the sight of him?

Exhausted from his intoxicated bout with the catmint, the orange cat leaped onto the bench and sprawled heavily across Dominic's lap. He stroked the sleek fur. He'd always had a gift for getting along with animals. His ability to ride even the wildest horses was legendary, and dogs and cats generally climbed all over him, as this one was doing. Surely he could also soothe a wild girl.

A day and a half passed without another sighting of Dominic's elusive quarry. To fill in some of the idle hours, he borrowed a set of estate maps Mrs. Marks found for him. After studying the layout of the various gardens, he drew a rough map small enough to carry with him, but it didn't bring him any closer to Lady Meriel.

As boredom set in, it occurred to Dominic that animal traps were usually baited with food, and what worked for rodents might work with a wild girl. The next afternoon he made his way through the gardens with a heavily laden basket in one hand.

There were easily two dozen specialized gardens of all sizes and shapes, ranging from a small butterfly garden to the large mock wilderness area where Lady Meriel had vanished. Yet vast though they were, the gardens covered less than a quarter of the park, and the park was only one corner of an estate that included a large home farm and five sizable tenant farms. He tried to suppress a pang at the knowledge that this splendid property would end up under the control of Kyle, who would eventually inherit vast estates of his own, yet had no great passion for the land.

Having come to a small garden that stepped down to a lily pond in several brick terraces, Dominic paused to consult his map. Where was the water garden? Ah, there. His destination was Lady Meriel's tree house, which Mrs. Rector had said was built in the center of the gardens. If he left the water garden by the right-hand path and wandered through an orchard of mixed fruits, he should find the tree.

A few minutes' walk brought him to a peaceful glade surrounding the largest oak he'd ever seen. Thick and tall and broad, the tree must be centuries old, and contained enough lumber to build a sizable sailing ship.

Even more impressive was the tree house nestled among the wide branches. Probably the structure had been built by Kamal, for it was styled like an Eastern palace. Easily a dozen feet square, the tree house featured a gilded onion dome roof and a tall, slim minaret. Painted a warm golden white and trimmed with green and gold traceries, it was the perfect abode for a young woman who looked like a fairy. The sheer whimsy of the structure made him want to laugh aloud.

Access was by a rope ladder that dropped through a hole in the floor. Mrs. Marks said that when the girl was inside, she usually pulled the ladder up behind her. Since there was no ladder visible, she must be in residence.

Proof of that came when a large canine head popped up alertly in a spot just below the tree house. Mrs. Marks said that the dog, a bitch called Roxana, followed Lady Meriel everywhere except into the tree house, paws not being well suited for rope ladders. Now the dog guarded her mistress's privacy.

Time to get to work. Ignoring Roxana's suspicious gaze, Dominic took a folded blanket off the basket and spread it on the grass in the center of the sunny glade. The uncovered basket released enticing aromas through the clearing. The Warfield cook had said that Lady Meriel hadn't come to the kitchen all day, so the girl was probably hungry. At Dominic's request, the cook had made some of the young mistress's favorite foods.

After settling on the blanket on crossed legs, Dominic dug into the basket. He started with a savory custard pie flavored with cheese, small pieces of smoky ham, and herbs from Meriel's own garden. Still warm from the oven, it smelled heavenly.

Though he'd been told often enough that the girl didn't understand anything that was said to her, surely she was capable of responding to tone of voice like a dog or a horse. In a voice pitched to carry easily without sounding threatening, he said, "Good afternoon, Lady Meriel. Would you care to dine with me?"

No response from the lady, but the dog

51

began to quiver with interest, the black nose twitching. Dominic sliced the pie into pieces and removed a narrow wedge. "Would you like something, too, Roxana?"

She leaped to her feet and padded over to Dominic. The beast was *large*. Trying not to think how easily a dog could rip out a sitting man's throat, Dominic tossed a chunk of pie to her. She snapped it from the air with a flash of long, sharp teeth. "Good dog!" He threw another piece.

After gulping the second morsel, the dog settled beside Dominic, all hostility forgotten as he scratched her floppy ears. Roxana was of no known breed, though he suspected some wolfhound because of her size. Her proportions were rather strange, but she seemed intelligent and good-natured. What more could one want in a dog?

Turning back to the basket, Dominic pulled out plates, mugs, napkins, and forks. Then he removed a stone jug. "I have some cider here. Would you care for some?"

He risked a glance up at the tree house. A small feminine silhouette was visible in the window. "There's fresh hot gingerbread, too. Perhaps you can smell it."

After pouring himself cider, he put a piece of the savory pie on one of the two plates he'd brought. Not having eaten since breakfast, he was hungry himself. After the first forkful, he sighed with satisfaction. The Warfield cook's crumbly pastry and well-flavored filling would not have disgraced the king's own table.

Abruptly a rope ladder rattled down from the tree house. The rungs were made of smooth wooden bars. They would make climbing easier than if the ladder was entirely rope, but Lady Meriel must still be more agile than the average female.

The ladder began swaying. Not wanting to frighten his quarry, he refrained from looking up, but he watched the ladder from the corner of his eye until a slender bare foot, rather dirty, appeared. He learned that when a female descended a rope ladder, a delightful amount of shapely ankle was exposed. Controlling his expression, he calmly cut another piece of pie and placed it on the other plate.

Then he turned toward her unhurriedly. Once more, he was struck by the power of her beauty. She seemed too fragile to have survived the savage loss of her parents and a barbaric captivity. But she hadn't survived, not really. All the potentials of her mind and spirit had been destroyed, leaving only a shadow of what might have been.

He leaned across the blanket and set the second plate on the edge nearest her, then poured another mug of cider. Lady Meriel had reached the ground and stood with one hand on the ladder as she looked in his direction without meeting his gaze. Her eyes were an extraordinary light, clear green. The eyes of a seer—or a madwoman.

It was clear that if he made one wrong move, she'd be up the tree like a squirrel. "I will never hurt you, Lady Meriel," he said softly. "You have my word on that."

Roxana got to her feet and pattered over to her mistress, tail wagging. Perhaps reassured by the dog's acceptance of the stranger, Meriel released the ladder and slowly crossed the glade toward Dominic. She moved with the grace of a young doe, her steps so delicate that her feet scarcely seemed to bend the grass.

He held his breath as she knelt by the blanket and lifted the plate. Her posture was poised and ready for flight, yet at the same time she was relaxed. Or perhaps the right word was tranquil. Despite her eccentric dress and bare feet, she seemed utterly at home. This garden was her kingdom.

Balancing her plate with one hand, she ate as neatly as any lady at a formal dinner. He watched, entranced, as straight white teeth sank into the warm cheesy pie. There was something intimate about sharing this meal, just the two of them. Breaking bread together was one of humankind's most ancient rituals.

He looked away, reminding himself that his job was to be unthreatening, not intimate. After uncorking a wide-mouthed jar of pickled onions, he set the container within her reach. She lifted it, giving him a chance to observe her hands. They were not the well-tended, useless hands of a lady, but strong and practical, with calluses caused by gardening work. More beautiful than if she soaked them in ass's milk every day.

Despite her dusty bare feet, overall she was clean and well groomed. The thick braid shone like polished new ivory, containing almost no tint of color. Her brows and lashes were just dark enough to delicately define her features, rather than making her appear washed out. With her hair pulled back, he saw that neatly centered on her lobes were small silver crescent moon earrings. He had the odd thought that an ancient priestess might have been similarly adorned.

Turning his attention to her clothing, he saw that her green tunic and skirt were made of a fine, smooth cotton that would rest gently on Lady Meriel's delicate skin. Embroidery decorated the tunic's neckline and sleeves. Remembering Mrs. Rector's protectiveness of Lady Meriel, he had a poignant vision of the older woman embroidering the garment as a quiet way to express affection for a girl who would not even notice what had been done.

Lady Meriel finished the savory pie. He set the baking dish near her so she could take more if she wished. She reached out, the loose sleeve falling away, and he saw a bracelet high on her wrist. No, not a bracelet. He was shocked to see that the rust red filigreed band was a tattoo. That must have been done to her during her Indian captivity.

He had a brief, horrible image of a child writhing with pain as adults held her down and marred that porcelain skin with needles. Was that when she lost her voice, screaming helplessly? Had there been other tortures?

Appalled at the thought, he dug into the basket for the gingerbread. The cook had mentioned several sweets that the girl liked, and he'd chosen this because the spicy scent would carry best. Besides, he liked gingerbread, too.

He took a piece for himself and topped it generously with clotted cream from another jar before setting cake and cream near Lady Meriel. Main meal finished, she helped herself to the gingerbread. She liked clotted cream as much as he did.

It was almost possible to believe she was normal, a young girl whose downcast gaze meant only shyness. But no normal girl, no matter how shy, would be so utterly indifferent to a companion. She never once met his eyes. If he spent much time around her, he would begin to wonder if he was invisible.

Though he doubted that she would understand, he said, "I'm going to be at Warfield for several weeks, Lady Meriel. I want to get to know you better."

Oblivious, she broke off a corner of the gingerbread and tossed it to Roxana. The dog seized the tidbit eagerly and approached her mistress for more. Lady Meriel caressed the large head and then offered more cake. As least she was aware of the dog, if not Dominic, he thought with mild exasperation.

Could she be deaf? No one had suggested the possibility, but it might explain her lack of responsiveness. He put two fingers in his mouth and gave a piercing whistle. Her head whipped toward him, then away again so quickly that he had no time to catch her glance. Still, she obviously wasn't deaf.

Try again. "The Warfield gardens are magnificent, the finest I've ever seen. I'd like to see them all. If you don't object, perhaps tomorrow I can accompany you as you do your work. I promise I won't get in the way. In fact, I can help. You're in charge, since they're your gardens, but I'm good at fetching and carrying and digging."

He stopped, realizing that even though he was using his brother's expression and inflections, the words were all wrong. Kyle wasn't lazy, but he would never volunteer to work like a laborer.

To hell with acting like Kyle. Meriel wouldn't know the difference, and Dominic must do something to ingratiate himself with her.

It occurred to him that she deserved to have a name for her suitor. Which name, though? A wife might call her husband by his Christian name, but it stuck in Dominic's craw to call himself Kyle. Better to use the name he and his brother had in common. If Kyle questioned that, Dominic could claim that he didn't want to teach the girl to recognize a title that would someday change from Maxwell to Wrexham. "I believe I was introduced to you as Lord Maxwell when I was here before, but you may think of me as Renbourne. It's my family name, and may someday be yours. May I call you Meriel, since we will be seeing much of each other?"

As expected, she did not object to the liberty of dropping her title. Meriel it would be.

He reached for the cider jug without noticing that she was doing the same. Their fingers collided. He felt an instant of shock, and she jerked her hand back as if scalded. He felt a perverse satisfaction. For a moment, at least, she had recognized his existence.

That recognition came at a cost. Smoothly she rose to her feet and crossed the glade to the ladder. He jumped up. "Wait, Meriel! Perhaps we could go for a walk. You could show me more of the gardens."

He might as well not have spoken. Swiftly she ascended the ladder, her full skirt rippling around her ankles. She disappeared into the square access hole, pulled up the ladder, then dropped a wooden hatch cover in place with solid finality.

His jaw clenched as he fought the impulse to climb the damned tree and go in a window after her. He was here to persuade, not coerce.

Mouth tight, he packed up the remains of the picnic. He supposed he'd made progress— but not enough.

Chapter 5

That night she dreamed of fire. Flames that scorched the sky, shouts of terror, screaming horses and humans. She awoke covered in perspiration, her body shaking. The nightmare came less often in recent years, but the terror never diminished.

Shivering, she threw off her blanket and fumbled her way across the tree house. It was late, after moonset, and very dark. She removed the hatch cover by touch and lowered the ladder. Roxana wakened below and whimpered a welcome.

Cautiously Meriel descended the swaying ladder. Earlier it had rained, and the night was cool and damp. She reached the ground, then wrapped herself around the dog's shaggy body. Roxana licked her face before settling down again contentedly.

In the dark and silence, the pulse of life around her was very clear. The oak was deep and strong and slow, this night only an instant in an existence measured in centuries. A lethal whir of wings, a sharp hunger, marked the passage of an owl seeking prey. Even the grass had a signature tone, light and swift and heedless in its uncounted numbers.

All her life, she had sensed the life forces around her. With humans, vital force often showed as a colored haze around the body, especially in dim rooms or when seen from the corner of an eye. Of the two ladies, Mrs. Rector was a soft, warm pink, Mrs. Marks a clear yellow except when she was irritated. Then her light darkened and faint orange streaks would show around her. Kamal radiated a pure blue that deepened when he spoke of spiritual matters, and the challenges of living well in an imperfect world. His light had guided her as truly as his words.

With Renbourne, she could see the glow of

his energy even in sunlight. His essence danced in a way that was at odds with his stern expression. Gold and scarlet shimmered about him, the clearest colors she'd ever seen. Sometimes she wondered what her own colors were, but it was impossible to tell, even by looking in a mirror.

Ashamed of having impulsively fled from Renbourne in the herb garden, she'd decided to accept his proffered food. Roxana liked him, and besides, she'd been hungry. She hadn't expected the impact of his nearness, and his touch. Her fingers curled involuntarily when she remembered that sparking energy.

He was unlike anyone else who had ever come to Warfield. She told herself that it was only because he was a young male, but that didn't explain tonight's restlessness, an empty feeling for which she had no name.

Mist was rising, and even with Roxana's warmth the ground was too cold and damp for rest. She stood and snapped her fingers. Obediently the dog rose and they made their way to the house. The night was alive with the stirring of nocturnal creatures busy about their business.

Though it wasn't the shortest route, she crossed the woodland for the pleasure of hearing the badgers at play, then wound through the moon garden. As a small child, the dimly remembered presence known as Papa had once laughingly said she had a cat's vision at night. Perhaps it was true. Certainly she had no trouble finding her way through even the deepest shadows.

They reached the house, where a small side door was her usual entrance and exit. She located the hidden key by touch and let herself in. Side by side, she and Roxana ascended the narrow, enclosed stairwell that led up to the corridor by her bedroom. Her fingertips skimmed the wall as Roxana's claws tapped hollowly on the bare wooden steps.

In her bedroom, a faint light from the window revealed a round shape on her bed. Ginger. The cat raised his head and gave a *mrrrrp* of welcome. Cold and tired, she slid under the covers without bothering to undress and curled around the cat. Roxana followed, settling on the foot of the bed with a canine sigh.

The emptiness didn't go away, but finally, warmed by her friends, she slept.

By luck, Dominic glanced out his window the next morning just as he finished dressing. Meriel and Roxana were disappearing in the direction of the garden sheds. According to Mrs. Marks, Meriel often met with Kamal there in the morning, presumably to commune in some strange way about what she wanted done. Anxious to catch up with her, he hurried downstairs and outside with no more than a wistful regret for the breakfast he was missing.

As he cut through the parterre, he thought about how everyone placidly accepted Meriel's comings and goings as if she were a privileged house pet. This whole household was organized around her condition, yet she was scarcely more than a will-o'-the-wisp.

But he understood now why she had never been turned over to a mental asylum. No rational human could want to see such a beautiful creature caged. Here she did no one any harm, and presumably enjoyed life in her own way.

Despite his haste, when he reached the garden sheds Kamal was alone. The Indian was sitting cross-legged on the ground outside the glass house, eyes closed and hands relaxed. Dominic hesitated, not wanting to disturb what might be a prayer.

Kamal's eyes opened. "Good morning, my lord," he said, unperturbed.

Remembering how Kamal had greeted him the day before, Dominic pressed his hands together in front of his chest and inclined his head. "Namaste, Kamal. Has Lady Meriel come this way?"

The older man got to his feet. "She works in the topiary garden this morning."

The topiary? That might be interesting. "Is there some way I might aid her?"

Kamal studied him shrewdly. "Only in menial tasks beneath my lord's dignity."

Dominic made an impatient gesture with one hand. "I am more concerned with spending time with the lady than with my dignity. How can I help?"

"She is trimming the yews," Kamal replied, approval in his dark eyes. "The clippings will need to be removed. If you are willing, there are sacks inside the shed."

Dominic started toward the shed indicated,

then paused. The tattoos on Kamal's cheeks appeared to have faded slightly. Was that possible? "Forgive my curiosity, but I wondered about the tattoos. They are very...striking. Unusual."

"Tattoos? Ah, the *mehndi*." Kamal held out his hands. The designs there also seemed slightly lighter than the day before. "They are painted on with henna. A custom in my native land. They wear off after a week or two."

"I see." Dominic said, glad the patterns had been achieved without painful tattooing. "You painted these on yourself?"

Kamal shook his head. "The young mistress did them."

"Lady Meriel?" Startled, Dominic looked more closely at the designs. Such intricate work must require a high level of skill. "Did you teach her how?"

"Aye. She had seen mehndi as a child in India. When she began to draw on herself with berry juice, I thought it best that she learn to use henna." Smiling a little, Kamal flexed one decorated hand. "She has now surpassed her teacher."

"I saw yesterday that she had what seemed to be a tattooed bracelet. Another of the"— he groped for the word—"mehndi?"

"Aye. She was in a playful mood."

Glad to relinquish the nightmare vision of a small girl being stabbed with needles, Dominic entered the shed. A pale spiny creature was curled on top of the stack of large burlap garden sacks. Bemused, he stepped from the shed and remarked, "There's a white hedgehog sleeping in here."

"The young mistress's pet, Snowball. Very rare, the white ones. She found him when he was injured and raised him in a cage. Now he lives free." Amusement glinted in Kamal's eyes. "His life is too good for him to wish to leave."

Dominic had a new mental image, this time of Meriel earnestly catching worms and grubs to feed a young hedgehog. This vision he liked. But how to get the sacks he needed without disturbing Snowball?

After due consideration, he collected all four corners of the top sack, transferred them to one hand, and hoisted the hedgehog while he yanked half a dozen sacks from the pile with his other hand. Then he lowered the top sack and flattened it back into place.

Startled awake, the little animal blinked pink eyes and briefly bristled its spines. Then it curled up again and went back to sleep.

Grinning, Dominic tossed the sacks over one shoulder and went in search of the topiary. The area was on the far side of the garden complex. His map showed that the inner gardens were like a series of rooms designed around a theme such as pond lilies or roses or herbs. Farther out were larger areas designed to give the eye constantly changing vistas. The topiary was such a place.

As he walked, he thought about the henna bracelet Meriel had painted on herself. Which wrist? He visualized her reaching, and saw that it was her right wrist. She must be left-handed to have painted that. Yes, she consistently favored her left hand.

Putting together the various things he'd been told about Kyle's intended bride, he realized that two different states were implied. One was idiocy, a complete lack of normal intelligence. The other was madness. Yet surely it required intelligence and skill to be a good gardener, tame animals, and paint those complex patterns. Her mind might work in unusual ways, but it definitely worked. So she was no idiot.

What did it mean to be mad? People tossed the term around casually, but he didn't really know what madness was. Frothing at the mouth, uncontrollable rages, and wildness were obvious signs of derangement, but Meriel exhibited none of these. Instead, she lived in a private world, incapable of human interaction. Maybe she was only a little mad and might be cured?

He needed to know more. Later he would talk to Meriel's chaperons, perhaps look in the library to see if there were any texts he could consult.

Dominic crested a gentle hill and looked down over a sweeping vista. To the left, he could see the river that bordered one edge of Warfield, and Castle Hill, topped with Norman ruins. The middle distance showed a quilt of fields and pastures marked by dark hedges. Nearer, the tall stone wall separated the park from the fields. The only sign of human life was a distant gardener patiently rolling turf with a wide stone roller.

His gaze dropped to the area just below, and he caught his breath. The hillside had been turned into a chessboard sculpted from living plants. The board was formed by alternating squares of grass, with half darker than the others. Topiary chess pieces caught a game in progress. Two types of dense evergreen were used, one dark green and the other much lighter, a green gold. Yew and variegated boxwood, Dominic guessed.

The distinctly different colors neatly divided the chess pieces into "black" and "white." Half a dozen pieces had been taken from the board and set in a cluster to one side. Black appeared to be winning.

A flicker of blue fabric appeared near the center of the chessboard. Guessing that none of the aging gardeners would wear such a color, he was about to descend the hill when he glimpsed a horse and rider jumping a hedge from the corner of his eye.

He turned for a closer look, and was startled to see that the leaping horse and rider were topiary, shaped of the same dark green yew as the hedge they were hurdling. In fact, there was a whole life-sized topiary hunt consisting of three riders and a small pack of hounds strung out across the grass as they dashed after a fleet, high-tailed fox.

Enchanted, he went to examine the nearest yew hound. It seemed to soar over the grass, front and back legs stretched out in a run. He'd never seen anything like it, for usually topiary was confined to geometric shapes like spirals and cubes and pyramids.

Inside the dense green leaves, he found a wicker form bent to the rough shape of a dog. Refinement was supplied by the careful trimming of the bush that had been trained around the armature. It must have taken years—decades—to achieve such perfection.

The hound had just been trimmed—clippings lay around it on the grass. He scooped them up and tossed them into a sack, then went in search of Lady Meriel, stopping long enough to collect the trimmings from the green fox.

The fox was heading straight into the collection of topiary chess pieces that had been "removed" from the game. He supposed it made sense, if one was a topiary fox.

As he neared the chessboard, he realized how large the pieces were. Even the pawns loomed over his head. The knights were shorter but magnificent, with broad horse heads and a suggestion of hooded eyes. There couldn't be finer topiary anywhere in Britain.

Some of the pieces were trimmed as sharply as marble, while others looked rather shaggy. Maintaining the shapes must take an immense amount of effort, especially during the spring growth season.

He was admiring the crenellated top of a rook when he heard a soft, lyrical sound coming from somewhere nearby. Not birdsong; perhaps it was some kind of musical instrument. One that sounded almost like a human voice.

Intrigued, he followed the music, moving quietly on the velvety grass. Then he emerged from between two pawns, and stopped dead in his tracks.

Lady Meriel was singing.

She stood with her back to him two squares away, trimming the white queen with a pair of clippers. Her slim form was clothed in a blue tunic and skirt much like what she'd worn the day before, but he scarcely noticed. She was *singing*!

He thought back and realized that no one had ever said she was mute, just that she didn't talk, which was not the same thing. Her voice was smooth and light, clearly used regularly, even if only to serenade shrubs. The tune had a wistful minor-key quality that made him think of a harpist he'd heard in Ireland. But she uttered no words, only that haunting ribbon of sound.

Deciding it was time to announce himself, he stepped forward. "Good morning, Meriel. I've come to help."

She used her shears to snip off a branchlet with lethal precision but didn't turn. Nonetheless, she knew he was there. He could tell by the subtle tensing of her shoulders. Less aloof, Roxana left her spot in the queen's shadow and loped over to get her head scratched before flopping again.

Meriel had trimmed several of the chess pieces in the area, so he gathered the clippings and bagged them as her song wove around him. Then he turned his attention to her again. He was amused to see that the queen's head was shaggy because Meriel couldn't reach high enough to trim it. Here was a way to make himself useful.

Several tools were piled by the black bishop, so he lifted a pair of long-handled pruning shears and moved to the far side of the white queen from Meriel. By stretching, he was just able to reach the tip and clip off a ragged sprout of box.

The singing stopped abruptly and Meriel whipped around the shrub, clippers held like a weapon. Her gaze shot to the top of the topiary queen.

"I've done no damage," he said mildly. "Even a useless gentleman can do this kind of work when the topiary shapes are so well defined."

Her gaze flicked over him so quickly that once again she managed to avoid meeting his eyes, but she seemed satisfied. Returning to her side of the shrub, she continued her trimming with sharp snaps of her clippers. No more singing, to his regret.

Since the day was warm and his coat made it hard to raise his arms over his head, he stripped off the garment and tossed it aside before resuming work. He took great pains with the top of the queen, sure there would be hell to pay with Lady Meriel if he damaged such an important piece.

He was so intent on doing the job right that he almost stumbled over Meriel as he worked his way around the shrub. Off balance with the effort of not stepping on her bare feet, he lurched and instinctively caught her elbow to steady himself. Everything seemed to stop—his movements, hers, the lazy breeze.

Everything but his heart, which suddenly accelerated.

He looked down at the crown of her head, where flaxen hair pulled back into the heavy braid that fell past her waist. She stood frozen, her gaze on his throat, but he could see a pulse beat in her jaw. A delicate film of perspiration sheened her pearly complexion.

Lord, she was small, her head barely reaching his chin. Yet not fragile, despite her slight build. There was wiry strength in the arm under his hand, and tension in her slim, elegant frame. What would he see if she raised those demurely downcast eyes—alarm, or anger?

"You're not used to being touched, are you?" He made himself release her arm. "Yet marriage involves touching of the most intimate kind. I wonder how you would react to that. With revulsion? Endurance? Or possibly pleasure?"

He expected her to draw away, perhaps even flee. Instead, she raised her left hand and touched his bare throat. His muscles spasmed under his skin in reaction to the light, almost caressing stroke of her fingers. He felt the faint roughness of calluses on her fingertips, heard their delicate rasp against his whiskers. Her intent exploration sent chills through him as she skimmed his throat and jaw, traced the outline of his ear.

At least, by God, she was aware of him.

"You have a voice, Meriel," he said softly. "Can't you use it to say yes or no? To speak my name?"

Abruptly she whirled away and stalked across the board to another chess piece, this time the black bishop. Definitely a stalk, not a walk.

He supposed that was her way of saying no.

Her hands shook so much that she cut too deeply, marring the smooth surface of the dark bishop. *His fault! In two short days, he had gone from being a creature with no more importance than a sparrow to being fully alive, as real as Kamal. Even the ladies lacked his vividness and texture.*

She made herself pause, slow her breathing, before she resumed clipping the bishop. Renbourne would go soon, for he was too much of the world to linger in so quiet a place. But until then, he would disturb her peace, for he was impossible to ignore.

At least he was capable of trimming a shrub without damaging it. She glanced across the board. His arms were lifted above his head to shape the top of the pale queen. The white shirt drew taut across his wide shoulders. Their breadth narrowed down sharply to his waist and hips, forming a triangle that pleased the eye. She gazed at him, enjoying his movements, until he finished and started to turn toward her.

Hastily she bent her head to the bishop again. There was no reason for her face to heat at the knowledge that she found pleasure in watching him. Every day she observed the bees and badgers, birds and butterflies, and the other creatures of Warfield. All life was lovely in its own way. He was simply one more beautiful beast, no different or more important than the others.

She told herself that...but she could not believe it.

Chapter 6

So far the voyage had been blessed with fine weather. Kyle was grateful for that, because Constancia was too frail to endure the bucking and twisting of stormy seas. This morning was calm, with just enough wind to fill the sails and drive them smoothly southward toward Spain.

He'd brought her outside to the private rear deck, where they could gaze at the following gulls. She reclined on a chaise, eyes closed but a faint smile on her face. Her skin was tanning from the sun, creating an illusion of health. The rich warm tones of her complexion had always been part of her allure.

"The light is different here," she murmured. "In England it is cool and blue. Here it is warmer. Full of reds and yellows."

She was right, he realized. Strange. He'd always yearned to travel, yet he was oblivious to the sights of this trip. All his concentration was on her.

In the same lazy tone, she said, "The girl in Shropshire who is to be your wife. What is she like?"

He'd scarcely thought of Warfield, and what was happening there. He tried to remember his impressions of Lady Meriel. "Small. Colorless." His mouth twisted without humor. "And very, very rich."

Constancia's eyes opened. "It sounds as if you do not like her."

"I scarcely know her. People like me are not supposed to have strong feelings about whom we marry. My life belongs to Wrexham." He tried to keep the bitterness from his voice, with little success.

"Nonsense. No one can make you wed against your will. Surely you should have at least some fondness for the girl who will be your wife." Constancia frowned. "Though I cannot imagine she will not notice when her current suitor becomes someone else at your next meeting. No twins are so identical that a future bride will not see the difference. Are you hoping she will become so angry she will refuse the marriage?"

"She won't notice." He looked away from Constancia, knowing he shouldn't say more. But the habit of honesty was impossible to break. "The girl isn't right in the head."

Constancia caught her breath, shocked. "Kyle, you are going to marry a fool or a madwoman? Surely you will do nothing so absurd!"

"Lady Meriel is neither. Merely...lost in her own world. Her uncle hopes that marriage may bring her more into normal life."

Constancia made an indescribable Spanish sound of disgust. "Perhaps you are the one who is mad, querido. To send the brother you despise to court a bride who is weak in the head! *Madre de Dios*, have you no concern for the rest of your life?"

He stalked to the railing, bracing himself on the polished wood as he stared at the shifting seas. When his father had first broached the subject of Lady Meriel, marriage had seemed endurable because he would always have Constancia. Then her illness had struck, and nothing else mattered.

Her voice gentling, Constancia asked, "Tell me of your brother, querido. You say he is irresponsible, and you never speak of him. Yet he is blood of your blood, flesh of your flesh. You shared the same womb. Surely he must be important to you."

"We probably had our first fight in our mother's womb," he said dryly. "The first, but certainly not the last."

"You have always been enemies?"

He watched a gull plunge straight into the sea in pursuit of prey. After a long silence, he said, "No. Sometimes we were friends. Good friends." He thought of nights curled up in the same bed, sharing stories and laughter. Dominic always knew how to laugh.... His gut twisted at the memories.

"What went wrong?" Her question was gentle as the sea breeze.

It was no accident that he'd never mentioned Dominic to Constancia. Even with her, the topic of his brother had been too painful to discuss. But the time for secrets was past. "As children we were always together, running wild at Dornleigh, studying with the same tutor. Sometimes we skirmished, but it was never important. The trouble started when we were sent to two different schools."

"That must have been difficult."

His hands tightened on the railing. He'd cried his first nights at Eton, until an older boy found out and taunted him in front of his classmates. Dominic had suffered no such problems at Rugby. He came home for the holidays bubbling with stories about his new life. Hurt that he no longer seemed important to his brother, Kyle withdrew into aloof silence, and their closeness suffered the first, fatal crack. "As the years passed, we had less and less in common. He had different friends, different interests."

"Was your brother jealous because you were the heir?"

"That was part of it." But resentment was too simple an explanation. Their father's steward had taught both boys what a gentleman needed to know about running an estate. Kyle had endured those lessons because he must. Dominic, damn him, had enjoyed them. He'd pelted the steward and bailiff with questions, learned everything he could about crop rotations and stock breeding. And he had seethed because Dornleigh would go to Kyle, who had no great affinity for the land. "I've sometimes thought that we were born to the wrong stations. He should have been the heir, not me. I would have enjoyed the freedom of being a younger son." He'd never admitted that to anyone.

"I see."

Knowing Constancia, she did see, perhaps more than Kyle did himself. There had been other problems between him and his brother. The tension had increased inexorably until the final rupture, shortly before they turned eighteen. After that, they seldom saw each other, and never again spoke intimately.

Their estrangement had taken place just before he met Constancia. Strange, how he'd never realized the significance of that. Dominic had left an aching hole in Kyle's life. What would have become of him if Constancia had not been there to fill the emptiness?

The sea was a strange place, he decided. It caused odd ideas to blow through a man's brain.

Chapter 7

Dominic and Meriel worked peacefully among the chess pieces until the sun was high in the sky. Then she gathered up her gardening tools in a handled canvas carrier and left without a glance in his direction, Roxana at her heels.

Abandoning his sacks of clippings to be collected by an undergardener, he grabbed his discarded coat and went in pursuit. As he fell into step beside her, he guessed that she was very aware of his presence, even though her gaze remained resolutely ahead. She had a lovely, delicate profile. In repose, her face looked pensive. A little remote, but not at all mad.

He took the tool carrier from her hand. She let him have it after an instant of resistance. Clearly she neither expected nor desired help. He said conversationally, "If you sing again, I'll whistle along with you. I'm quite a good whistler."

No response. He began to whistle anyhow, choosing the old ballad "Barbara Allen" because the minor-key tune reminded him of Meriel's singing. She darted a swift glance at him, turning away before he could catch her gaze. Still, it was a response. Congreve was right—music had charms to soothe a savage breast. Not that Meriel was exactly savage— but neither was she civilized.

She chose a route he hadn't seen before, following a narrow gorge with a brook at the bottom. Shaded by tall trees, the path ran along the stream bank between drifts of late spring flowers. He stopped whistling to listen to the sounds of water trickling over stones and into pools. On a hot day, this little glen would be a perfect retreat.

"A lovely place," he remarked. "Too perfect to be quite natural. The original gorge was carefully improved, I presume? You are mistress of the most remarkable gardens I've ever seen, Lady Meriel. This estate should have been called the Elysian Fields. That's the abode of the blessed dead in Greek mythology. Did anyone ever read Greek myths to you when you were a child? The Greeks were a quarrelsome lot, but they left us wonderful stories."

He had a brief flash of memory: he and Kyle acting out the Trojan War, when they were seven or eight. His brother was noble Ajax, while Dominic chose to be wily Odysseus. They'd been too young to recognize how characteristic their choices were.

Shaking off the image, he continued, "Shall I read to you in the evening, Meriel? I would enjoy that." He liked the idea of bathing her in the great tales of classical literature. Perhaps such a flow of words would make a connection in her mind that would help bring her back to the world.

He glanced again at that impassive, perfectly carved profile. Perhaps not; maybe the damage done to her as a child could never be repaired. It was so damned *unfair*.

No longer in the mood for a one-sided conversation, he fell silent until they reached the garden sheds. She went straight for the glass house. Inside, Kamal was tending to the pineapple plants. All the best houses grew pineapples to impress guests; Dornleigh had devoted half a glass house to their cultivation.

Kamal glanced up casually at their entrance, his brows rising a little at the sight of Dominic. He had probably assumed that a pampered aristocrat wouldn't last long trimming shrubs. Inclining his head respectfully, he said to Meriel, "You should eat something before going off again, milady."

As Meriel gazed at him expectantly, the Indian moved down the aisle until he found a pineapple that pleased him. Then he pulled a glittering dagger from a sheath mostly concealed by the sash at his waist and harvested the pineapple from its spiky growth. After trimming off the bristly brown skin, he laid the fruit on a clean cutting board. A dozen wicked slashes of the dagger sliced the pineapple from its tough core into eating wedges. As he watched the expert knife work, Dominic made a mental note never to provoke Kamal's temper.

With a courtly bow, the Indian offered the board of sliced fruit, juice oozing over the edges. "My lady. My lord."

Meriel took a wedge and bit neatly into the golden flesh with small white teeth. Dominic took a piece also, but paused before eating. "Will you join us, Kamal?" When the Indian hesitated, Dominic added, "Our Bible says that the oxen who tread out the grain should not be prevented from tasting the products of their labor. Surely that is even more true for a master gardener who grows such beautiful fruit."

"You are gracious, my lord." Kamal set

the board on the adjacent workbench and took a slice of pineapple. Though his words were flawlessly polite, there might have been an edge of irony in his tone. The Indian didn't seem like a man whose thoughts would ever be simple ones.

Dominic bit into his wedge of pineapple. It was the finest he'd ever eaten, tart and sweet and luscious with juice. If he were ten years old, he would have moaned with pleasure. He barely refrained from doing so even at his advanced age. "Superb, Kamal."

Apart from that comment, the three of them consumed the pineapple in silence. Dominic's London friends would have laughed at the sight of him eating in a glass house with a foreign servant and a beautiful mad girl. Yet though it was hardly a normal luncheon, he enjoyed it immensely.

After finishing her portion, Meriel turned and headed toward the far end of the glass house. Dominic asked, "Do you know what she plans on doing this afternoon?"

Kamal swallowed his last bite of pineapple. "No, my lord, though often she prefers a different kind of task from what she did in the morning."

So probably no more pruning today. Dominic went after Meriel, who had halted by the pump in the far corner of the glass house. Seeing that it was awkward to work the handle and wash at the same time, Dominic took over the pumping, his hands bracketing her much smaller one.

Accepting his help, Meriel washed and dried her hands on a shabby but clean towel that hung from a nail. She started to turn away, then hesitated as if a thought had struck her. Taking hold of the handle, she began to pump. He realized that she was returning the favor so he could wash his own hands. Oddly touched, he held them under the water and rinsed away juice and yew stains. "Thank you, Meriel."

When he pulled his clean hands from the stream of water, she walked away with her customary lack of ceremony. Like a cat, she never looked back.

Her first stop was in the shed that her hedgehog called home. As she knelt beside the pile of burlap sacks, Snowball woke up and rolled onto his back so she could stroke his tender stomach. Dominic watched with amusement from the doorway. He hadn't known that hedgehogs could smile. Well, he would himself if those strong, well-shaped hands were stroking his belly.

The thought was a disturbing one, made more so when a lock of her glossy blond hair fell forward across the little animal. The pale strands were almost the same shade as Snowball's albino spines. Would Kyle enjoy watching her play with a pet? Probably not. His twin was too restless, too impatient, for such small pleasures.

Meriel gave the hedgehog a last caress and rose gracefully from her kneeling position. Brushing by Dominic in the doorway as if he were invisible, she left the shed and headed toward the house.

Falling into step beside her, he observed, "You have a gift for dealing with animals. Rather like Saint Francis of Assisi. I don't suppose anyone ever told you about him, Francis being a Catholic saint, but I've always thought he'd be an interesting fellow to meet. They say wild creatures came to his hand, as tame as Roxana. He called them his brothers and sisters."

Dominic had a sudden memory of a painting he'd once seen that showed Saint Francis sitting in a clearing, birds on his shoulder, foxes and deer and other beasts gathered around him. On the saint's face was an expression as unworldly as Meriel's. Maybe saints and madmen were close kin?

He continued his idle talk, telling his companion everything he knew about St. Francis. Though she never turned her head, he sensed that she was listening, though perhaps only to the rhythm of his voice rather than his words.

As they neared the stable block, he realized that he ought to exercise Kyle's horse. "Would you like to meet Pegasus, Meriel?"

He touched her elbow to guide her into the open stable doors. She balked and almost pulled away. Guessing that she was afraid of horses, he said coaxingly, "He's a splendid beast, named for a winged horse of Greek legend."

With dragging feet, she accompanied him into the dim stable. Keeping a close eye on her, he asked, "Do you ride?" He scanned the unimpressive Warfield horses. "No, I don't suppose so. There isn't a decent riding hack here. Watch your step, now. Stables can be hazardous for bare feet."

Pegasus stuck his head out of a box stall and whinnied for attention. As Meriel stopped beyond biting distance, Dominic greeted the horse, stroking the silky nose and promising a ride. He glanced at his companion. "He won't harm you."

The low light made it hard to read her expression, but her posture indicated that she was on the verge of bolting. "You love animals, and they love you," he said softly. "Pegasus is a fine fellow, and he'd like to meet you."

Step by hesitant step, she moved forward. Her face showed not exactly fear, but deep reluctance. He moved back, allowing her to approach her own way. Luckily, the horse was extremely good-tempered.

Pegasus whuffled curiously, stretching out his neck toward Meriel. She tensed, then slowly raised her left hand and touched the white diamond on the horse's dark forehead. Against Pegasus's massive bulk, she looked pale and terribly fragile.

The horse nudged her shoulder enthusiastically. Even though the force of the movement almost knocked Meriel over, the tension eased from her body. Her other hand lifted to stroke the satiny neck.

Dominic exhaled with relief. Horse and

girl were going to be friends. Pegasus looked as happy under her touch as Snowball and Roxana did.

"Would you like to ride Pegasus?" When her hand stilled, he said, "With me, not on your own. I promise you'll be safe."

After a long, motionless interval, she closed her eyes and rested her forehead against the horse's neck, the black mane mingling with her own pale hair. Deciding that was a yes, Dominic said, "Very well, we'll take him out."

She moved away as he led the horse from the stall and saddled up. Pegasus almost danced with anticipation as Dominic took him outdoors. Glancing at Meriel, he said, "Keep clear when I first mount him. He'll be frisky from the lack of exercise."

Frisky was an understatement. As soon as Dominic swung into the saddle, Pegasus leaped exuberantly into the air. Dominic barely managed to clamp his legs around the horse's barrel in time to prevent himself from sailing across the stable yard. Perhaps that would have amused Meriel, but he had too much male pride to want that to happen in front of a pretty girl.

For several lively minutes, Pegasus worked off his high spirits in a series of bucks, twists, and kicks. Though there wasn't a mean bone in his body, he wasn't above testing his rider. Both of them enjoyed the process immensely until Dominic made it clear that it was time for the horse to behave.

84

Grinning, he brought Pegasus to a demure halt facing Meriel. It was going to be hard to return the horse to his brother. Maybe Kyle would be willing to sell? Probably not, and the price would surely be a year of Dominic's allowance.

During his bout with the horse, Meriel flattened herself against the stone wall of the stable, Roxana protectively close. She probably expected Dominic to get his brains dashed out on the cobbles. He wondered if she would care.

Collecting himself as he had collected the horse, he said calmly, "He's ready to accept a lady, Meriel. Come." He extended his hand.

He wouldn't have bet a ha'penny on his chances of luring her onto the horse, but she moved forward slowly, keeping a wary eye on Pegasus's iron-shod feet.

She paused an arm's length away, and her throat worked as she swallowed hard. Swiftly, as if wanting to act before she could change her mind, she took Dominic's hand and set her bare foot on his boot just in front of the stirrup. Smoothly he lifted, and she swung up behind him like thistledown. She settled down astride, her legs gripping the horse just behind his, and locked her slim arms around his waist.

He glanced down and saw that her leg was bared to just above the knee. The sight combined with the warm pressure of her body sent a dangerously erotic charge through him. This position was entirely too intimate.

Damning himself for his thoughts, he said, "You'll find that Warfield looks different from the back of a horse."

He set Pegasus in motion, starting with a walk. Meriel was pressed against him so tensely that he could feel how little she wore under her tunic and skirt. And she was definitely woman, not girl....

Keeping his gaze firmly ahead, he directed Pegasus around the house and into the long, grassy driveway, Roxana following. Pegasus's paces were smooth as silk, so gradually Meriel's grip eased. When he thought she was ready, he said, "We're going to change to a trot, so prepare for a different motion."

Did she understand and tighten her hold again? He wasn't sure, but she stayed on easily enough. Since trotting wasn't particularly comfortable for someone without stirrups, after a couple of minutes he warned, "We're going into a canter now."

He collected the horse, then shifted his weight forward and signaled the change of pace. Pegasus stretched gratefully into a long, smooth canter, flying across the green turf at a speed that matched the gallop of a lesser beast. They swept down the driveway, the trees blurring and the wind blowing Dominic's hair back.

Behind him, Meriel laughed with sheer exhilaration, a sound like singing bells. He'd never even seen her smile. His heart leaped in response. He wanted to sweep her into his arms, share the exuberance of speed and joy.

A good thing they were on horseback! She wasn't his to hug. She wasn't even Kyle's, not yet. Perhaps she never would be. Yet her delight was perilously alluring.

They were nearing the iron gates of the estate. He slowed Pegasus a little and said over his shoulder, "Since the day is so fine, I'll take you into the village...."

She gave a horrified cry, then released his waist and leaped from the moving horse.

Appalled, he reined in Pegasus and whirled around. She'd hit the ground and was rolling across the grass in a flurry of skirts and bare legs. He jumped from the horse, fearing she might have broken bones or worse. Before he could reach her, she scrambled up and darted through the trees that lined the drive.

Lashing his reins around a branch, he started after her. "Meriel, wait!"

Suddenly Roxana was growling in front of him, teeth bared. He stopped dead. The dog liked him, but it was clear she'd rip his throat out if he threatened her mistress.

He drew a deep breath, reminding himself that Meriel couldn't move so fast if she were hurt. Already she'd vanished into the park, her grass-stained garments blending with the shrubs and trees.

Was it mad for her to panic at the thought of leaving Warfield? Perhaps not, since the estate had been her haven since she was a small child.

But he wished to hell that someone had warned him.

Chapter 8

Dominic woke at dawn the next morning, pulled from a dream of flying through the sky on a winged horse while clasped by a silver-haired maiden who laughed like singing bells. In real life, he'd had no such luck. After the unfortunate end to their ride, Meriel had vanished for the rest of the day.

So much for his suggestion that he read Greek legends to her in the evening. The idea conjured up pleasant domestic images of sitting by a fire, Meriel listening dreamily while he shared some of his favorite stories with her. Maybe poetry, too.

He'd be better off reading to her cat. At least Ginger enjoyed coming in from the rain and sleeping by a warm fire. Lord only knew where Meriel had spent the night. He hoped she hadn't ended up in some damp, miserable hideaway.

The thought of her shivering and alone wrecked any chance of returning to sleep. He rose and went to the washstand to splash cold water in his face. As he dried himself, he glanced out the window. A thick, pearly mist covered the landscape. Though the sun must be up, he could barely see the patterns of the parterre below his window.

His eyes narrowed as he saw a human form moving through the parterre away from the house. Meriel. He was glad to see that she'd probably spent the night dry and warm inside.

But where the devil was she going at this hour? He dragged on clothing with a carelessness that would have appalled Morrison, then raced downstairs and outside into the foggy dawn.

She'd already vanished, so he continued in the direction he'd seen her going. Within a couple of minutes, he spotted her slim form. He slowed to match her pace, wondering what he hoped to achieve by this pursuit. Forgiveness for having frightened her into panicked flight the day before? She might have already forgotten the incident.

Then again, she might have become so wary that she'd never come near him again, which would doom his arrangement with Kyle. He tried to visualize himself as master of Bradshaw Manor, but the image wouldn't come. Maybe he'd botched this courtship beyond repair.

He felt oddly ambivalent about the possibility. Much as he wanted Bradshaw Manor, he was growing increasingly uncomfortable with his role. Meriel deserved better than a shabby deception. She deserved a man who cared about her, not one with so little interest in marriage that he wouldn't even court his own bride. Oh, Kyle would never hurt an innocent. He would just ignore the girl. He'd never take the time to learn what was rare and special about her.

Dominic spent a minute thinking about everything he hated about his brother before he forced his mind into more useful channels. Meriel had seemed to enjoy riding. Might she be capable of managing a horse on her own? Though her mind wasn't normal, she had her own kind of intelligence. Enough, perhaps, to master riding if she wished to.

He was beginning to suspect that she might be capable of doing far more than her guardians realized. In their desire to protect the girl, they had removed the challenges that might encourage growth.

Meriel had almost vanished, so he quickened his pace. Though she seemed unhurried, she covered the ground swiftly for someone so diminutive. It would be easy to lose her in the fog.

The mists reminded him of boyhood visits to Scotland, at his father's hunting box. He and Kyle had learned to stalk deer across the moors with the earl's ghillie, an ancient laconic Scot. Dominic had been a better tracker, with an ability to sense the deer's movements that had impressed even Auld Donald. But he'd had no stomach for shooting. The deer had been too beautiful to destroy.

Kyle had taken no pleasure in killing, but unlike Dominic, he had never balked. A first-rate marksman, he would coolly drop his prey without a flicker of visible remorse. The Earl of Wrexham had been proud of his heir.

Today Auld Donald's training stood Dominic in good stead, since Meriel was elusive even by the standards of shy Scottish deer. With her pale hair and flowing garments, he might have thought her a ghost if he hadn't known better.

They'd long since left the cultivated gardens, and the thickening fog implied they were approaching the river. The path began to climb at an angle that became steeper and steeper. He had to watch his footing, but he looked up regularly to check that he hadn't lost sight of his quarry.

He was starting to pant—how could a slip of a girl set such a pace on a hill this steep?—when he glanced up. He stopped dead, staring. The battlemented stone walls of a medieval castle loomed above, as ominous as a Gothic novel. An involuntary shiver spiked through him. The estate map had marked the site as "Norman ruins," but there was no hint that so much of the castle was still standing. The place was downright eerie.

Meriel passed through a gateway in the high outer wall. Once massive wooden doors had filled the space, but now tendrils of mist curled around the stonework. He paused, unsure whether he should follow her into a confined space where she could probably spot him easily.

But he hadn't come this far to stop now. Silent as the fog, he passed through the empty gateway into the ancient castle.

She'd known instantly who followed her. His energy was like a candle in the mist, vivid and distinctive. Her mouth tightened. She should have brought Roxana, who would have been happy to block his way. But Roxana was old and the damp hurt her bones, so Meriel had left her to sleep.

She loved the magic of the mist, the way it transformed the familiar landscape into something rare and strange. She might almost have been alone at the dawn of time—except for the persistent man behind her. Losing him would not be difficult. But a better idea struck when she thought how alarmed he'd been at her escape from his horse. She would give him something to worry about!

As she climbed the familiar path to the old castle, her mind's eye envisioned the moat full of water and home to swans. Prancing horses and ghostly pennons, ladies in flowing velvet and lords scarred in fierce, primitive battles. So vivid were the images that she wondered if she'd lived in the castle during its heyday. Hiral, her Hindu nurse, had said people were born again and again, learning lessons and growing in spirit through the ages. Meriel more than half believed her nurse's words, for surely the ties that bound her to Warfield had not been forged in a single lifetime.

Silently she said a prayer for Hiral, who had died in the massacre at Alwari. Her gentle nurse deserved to be reborn into a life of kindness and comfort.

Ordinarily Meriel went first to the roofless, hollow shell of the keep, but today she cut across the sheep-grazed bailey to the stone steps that led to the battlements. As she began to climb, she raised her voice in an eerie, wordless funeral song that she'd heard in India. Her voice echoed from the stones, uncanny as the cry of a lost soul.

She reached the wall walk and gazed across the river. On a clear day the hills of Wales were easily visible. This morning she could barely see the rushing waters far below as the currents swirled around the sheer cliffs that surrounded the castle on three sides. Her ancestor, Adrian of Warfield, had chosen well when he built his fortress here. Though attacked on several occasions, Warfield Castle had never been conquered.

Still singing, she drifted along the wall walk, avoiding the occasional crumbling stones, until she reached her destination. As her song rose to a crescendo, she climbed up into an embrasure. A faint breeze curled around her, lifting strands of her hair. The rising wind and warming sun would soon dissolve the mist.

She looked straight down the cliff, her body swaying to the rhythm of her song, her loose garments billowing about her. The stone was cold beneath her bare feet.

Then, as a voice shouted in horror behind her, she stepped into the air.

"Meriel! *Meriel!*" *Heart pounding in terror, Dominic bolted up the stone steps three at a time, shouting as if his voice could halt her suicidal plunge from the wall.*

He raced to the spot where she had jumped and peered over the battlements. The river was far, far below. Surely no one could survive such a fall, but still he scanned the waters, hoping for some sign of her. Nothing.

He swayed dizzily, wanting to vomit, as he fought the impulse to dive in after her. Not to save her—it was too late for that—but as penance for having driven an innocent to a horrific end. Meriel had lived here in peace for many years, until he arrived and destroyed whatever fragile restraints guarded her mind. He had begun to think of her as a fairly normal girl who merely had some odd quirks. Because of his stupidity, his lack of understanding, her broken body was being battered by the icy currents far below.

Then a flicker of movement caught his eye to his right, at the far end of the castle wall. He turned his head and stared. Green fabric? Wondering if his imagination was playing tricks, he leaned out the embrasure and looked straight down.

He'd thought the castle wall stood right on the cliff edge, but in this area there were several feet of margin between wall and cliff. Directly below him, centuries of gentle decay had caused earth and greenery to accumulate into a narrow shelf that rose to within eight or ten feet of the bottom of the embrasure. If someone dropped down to that shelf, it would be easy to edge along the base of the castle wall to safety.

He squinted and saw a faint impression of small bare feet in the damp soil. She was safe. *Safe.* He sagged against the wall, weak with relief.

Relief was swiftly followed by outrage. The little witch had deliberately tried to scare him out of his wits! He was as sure of that fact as he was of his own name. Maybe she was punishing him for his thoughtless attempt to take her outside Warfield.

Too angry for caution, he stepped from the wall and dropped onto the ledge. He landed hard, and the earth crumbled under his weight. He began to fall, and for a horrifying instant he knew he was doomed.

A wild swing of his hand caught a stout, wind-shaped shrub barely in time to save him. He clung to the gnarled branches, shaking. Meriel had probably landed more lightly, and she must know this castle like the back of her hand. Even so her trick had been damned dangerous. Maybe she didn't understand the peril of what she had done. He simply had no idea how that crooked little mind worked.

When his nerves had recovered, he flattened his back against the wall and began to inch his way along the cliff after Meriel. She'd had her fun, but by God, if she thought she'd lost him, she had better think again.

Chapter 9

Concealed in a clump of shrubs by the faint depression of the old moat, Meriel waited without impatience for Renbourne to appear. With most of her attention on the main gate, she almost missed seeing him emerge from behind the castle wall by the same route she had used. Foolish man! He could have got himself killed trying to follow her.

Still, he was clever to realize so quickly what she had done. Once she'd played the same trick on a disagreeable physician who had been dogging her steps to observe her madness. The dolt came tearing out of the castle, screaming that the river must be dredged. The ladies had sent him away after that incident.

Expression furious, Renbourne stormed down the hill toward her hiding place. Smiling, she slid away, taking care to stay out of his sight.

At the base of the hill she entered a broad belt of woodlands, since the fog wouldn't offer concealment much longer. Eventually she'd work her way back to the house for some food, but for now she was content to follow a favorite path through the woods, enjoying the chorus of birdsong.

She was in the most densely treed area when she heard another sound, low and filled with pain. She paused, frowning. The sound came again, a rough noise between a growl and a whimper. Somewhere nearby an animal was suffering.

She followed the sounds to a small clearing. A pair of foxes were there, the dog fox pacing anxiously around a whimpering vixen whose forepaw was caught in a sharp-toothed metal trap. Pure rage blazed through Meriel at the sight. *Poachers.*

Earlier in the spring she'd seen this pair of foxes at their courtship play, and her throat had tightened at the sight of their mutual enchantment. Now they were raising a litter of cubs nearby. In a careless moment the vixen had probably sprung a concealed trap that had been set for a hare. She lay on her side, panting, the vertical pupils of her eyes wide with pain and shock. Her right forepaw was a bloody mess.

Setting aside her fury in favor of more immediate concerns, Meriel stepped into the clearing. The dog fox gave a high sharp bark and retreated, though she guessed that he would not go far. Slowly she moved toward the vixen, humming to soothe the injured animal. To no avail; when Meriel stretched out a hand, the fox snapped viciously, her plumy tail lashing the ground.

Meriel snatched back her hand. Usually the wild creatures of Warfield were tolerant of her presence, but the vixen was in so much pain that she might be dangerous.

Twigs cracked nearby. Renbourne? No, his footsteps were lighter. Guessing that the poacher was coming, Meriel faded into concealment on the far side of the clearing.

A few moments later a roughly dressed youth with an empty game bag slung over his shoulder emerged from the shrubbery, his gaze going to the trap. A poacher, on *her* land, killing and maiming the creatures entrusted to her care!

Meriel gasped when he pulled a knife from a sheathe. He was going to cut the vixen's throat.

Screaming with rage, she sprang to her feet and launched herself at the intruder.

If not for Dominic's tracking skill, he never would have found Meriel's trail. She moved over the landscape as lightly as the retreating mists. But here and there she left flattened grass or a trace of footprint, and he'd catch up with her soon.

Then what? He was tempted to spank her, but he doubted that was appropriate for a young lady of twenty-three. Even one with a deplorable sense of humor.

His heart congealed when a blood-chilling female scream pierced the woodland air. This was no mock suicide, but a cry of genuine disaster. He broke into a run, wondering what could threaten her. Surely there were no dangerous animals in the park.

He should have remembered that the most dangerous beast was man. Bursting into a small clearing, he saw Meriel lying on the turf and a strange man on top of her, both of them struggling frantically. A rage unlike anything he'd ever known blazed through him. "You *bastard*!"

He dived into the fray and yanked the intruder off Meriel. Then he spun the man around and knocked him to the ground with one furious blow to the jaw. Dominic stood over him, fists clenched as he fought the desire to kick the rapist to a bloody pulp. "What kind of beast would assault a helpless girl?"

"Helpless!" the man protested in a thick Shropshire accent. Bleeding marks on his face showed where Meriel's nails had connected. "'Twas her that came after me! I'm just tryin' to keep her from scratchin' my eyes out."

Dominic glanced at Meriel, who'd risen from the ground. She did not look like a delicate maiden who had just been attacked by a rapist. Narrow-eyed and self-possessed, she watched the stranger with an expression as feral as a wolf's.

A quick scan revealed a trapped fox, a dropped skinning knife, and a game bag stained with dried blood from past kills. "A poacher," Dominic said with disgust.

The man lurched to his feet. Meriel instantly sprang, swinging a sharpened stick at his face. Dominic caught her in midleap, pulling her hard against him. Her small body was taut with furious strength. Gods above, to think he'd begun to imagine she was more or less normal! If this was an example of the tantrums Mrs. Rector had mentioned, no wonder the girl was thought mad. She was genuinely dangerous.

But her violence was not random, for she didn't turn on him when he grabbed her. He gave silent thanks. Subduing the little hellcat without one of them being hurt would be difficult. Luckily she fell still, glaring at the poacher with lethal intensity.

Seeing that the intruder was on the verge of flight, Dominic said dryly, "Stay put or I'll turn her loose, and she's fast. Very fast."

Watching Meriel warily, the man—or boy, really, he couldn't be more than seventeen, and skinny at that—said, "I wouldn't hurt the young miss. 'Tis known she's not right in her head." He rubbed his bleeding cheek. "She came after me like...like..."

"Like an avenging angel?" Hoping that Meriel would behave, Dominic released her before he became too distracted by the feel of her body against his. "No need to attack him, Lady Meriel. The law can handle a poacher. Seven years of transportation. New South Wales, I should imagine. Or maybe Van Diemen's Land."

The poacher turned white. "Please, sir, I meant no harm. What are a few more hares to a lord like you? You don't need them. Nor does she, with a fortune to last a thousand lifetimes." He bit his lip, looking very young. "If I'm transported, my mam and the little 'uns will starve. It's been hard since my pa died. There's no work."

Dominic's anger began to fade. He'd never approved of the law that made it a major crime for a landless man to take small game for the cooking pot. "I think Lady Meriel's fury stemmed from the fact that you hurt that fox, and to what purpose? Foxes are vermin, not game animals."

"If you're hungry enough, a fox isn't bad eating," the boy said bitterly. "Though a hare would've been better."

Dominic studied the boy's bony face and shabby, outgrown clothing. Such stark need put his own situation into perspective. He might be a younger son with no expectations, but he'd never missed any meals.

He dug into his pocket, hoping he had some money with him. Finding a coin, he pulled it out and tossed it to the boy. "Take this and buy food for your family. And if you value your freedom, don't ever set foot in Warfield Park again."

The boy gasped as he caught the gold sovereign, but Meriel flashed Dominic a darkling look. Tersely he said, "It's hard to condemn a man for trying to feed his family."

Perhaps she understood. Though she shifted rebelliously from foot to foot, she didn't make another move toward the poacher.

"Th-thank you, sir," the boy stammered, still staring at the coin. It was quite possible he'd never held a sovereign in his life.

Dominic frowned. A piece of gold could feed a family for a few days or even weeks, but it wasn't a permanent solution. "Tell me your name. I'm merely a guest at Warfield, so I can't make any promises. However, if you think a job would keep you from poaching, I'll ask the steward of the home farm if he needs laborers."

"Oh, sir!" The boy looked stunned. "I'll do any honest work."

A laborer made little enough, but at least the boy wouldn't risk being transported and leaving his mother with a cottage full of starving children. Dominic bent and picked up the fallen game bag and knife. "You can take these, but the trap stays here."

The boy nodded with resignation. There was no way he could use the trap legally; in fact, he could be arrested and convicted of poaching if he was even caught carrying the wretched thing. "Thank you, sir. My name is Jem Brown."

"Jem Brown. Very well, the day after tomorrow, present yourself to the Warfield steward. I'll have talked to him by then. Now go." Dominic donned the fierce scowl he'd learned during his brief career as a cavalry officer. "And don't forget what I said about staying out of the park."

Jem darted away before Dominic could change his mind. Meriel made a sound like a hissing cat as she watched him go. It would have been funny, if her behavior didn't underline how far she was from normal.

Putting aside that painful thought, he said, "It's time to see what we can do for that poor vixen. Just a moment."

He had passed a small brook on his way to the clearing, so he backtracked and soaked his handkerchief in the water. Then he returned to the trapped fox. Meriel crouched near the animal, concern in every line of her body.

The fox growled when Dominic knelt beside it. Knowing this would be harder than physicking a distressed horse or dog, he looked the vixen in the eyes as he mentally projected calm and good intentions. That he was a friend.

"There, there, old girl," he said softly. "Let's get you free. Then we can look at that leg. No need to worry. I used to think about becoming a veterinary surgeon, you know. I followed the Dornleigh farrier and the cowman and the shepherds around whenever I could, learning how to treat horses and cows and sheep. My father would have died of an apoplexy if I'd chosen to follow such a low trade, though."

The talk was mostly to soothe the fox with his tone of voice. He remembered just in time that he shouldn't say anything that would indicate he wasn't Kyle. While becoming a veterinary surgeon might be appalling in a younger son, it would be quite unthinkable for the heir to Wrexham.

Rather than speak more about his onetime ambitions, Dominic switched to talking about the fox—how splendid her white-tipped tail, how beautiful her cubs must be. When he thought she was calm enough, he laid an experimental hand on the thick, springy reddish fur of her shoulder. She quivered a little, but accepted his touch.

He turned his attention to the trap. The Dornleigh gamekeeper sometimes used traps to keep foxes from destroying the eggs of nesting game birds, but Dominic had never handled one. Wicked metal teeth clamped on the vixen's foreleg, with the tension supplied by a flat steel spring by the hinge.

Once he'd puzzled out how it worked, he rose and stepped on the spring. The metal jaw opened, and Meriel gently pulled the injured forepaw free.

"Just a little longer. Then you can go home to your cubs," Dominic murmured as he let the trap snap shut. He hoped he was telling the truth; if the injury was too severe, it might be kinder to destroy the poor beast.

Kneeling again, he used his wet handkerchief to carefully clean the damaged leg. He could sense Meriel's amazement that the vixen allowed the handling, but he didn't glance at her. All his attention was on the fox, whose sides heaved with distress.

After he'd washed away the crusted blood, he said with relief, "You're in luck, old girl. No bones broken, no tendons cut."

There was still some sluggish bleeding. If he were working on a lacerated horse or dog, he would apply salve and a bandage. He doubted that would work here, though. The vixen would probably gnaw at the bandage, possibly worsening the damage. "Follow your instincts, Madame Fox."

The vixen bent her head and a rough tongue came out to lick the wound. After several minutes of lapping, the ooze of blood had almost stopped.

"Are you ready to go home now?" he asked softly.

Shakily the vixen got to her feet. A sharp vulpine bark sounded from the edge of the clearing. The vixen's head shot up and her ears pricked. Then she bounded away to join her anxious mate. Though she favored the injured paw, she moved well. The dog fox gave a leap of joy before escorting his lady into the woods.

104

Dominic sat back on his heels, touched by the sight. "I think she'll recover. If you know where her den is, though, you might want to leave food nearby for a few days, to help the family out until she's in better shape."

He looked at Meriel, still crouched a yard away. She was gazing after the foxes, wearing an expression of profound gladness.

Then her head swung around, and for the first time she looked full into his face. He caught his breath, stunned by the depths and complexity visible in her clear green eyes. He'd thought her simple, he'd thought her mad, and from the beginning, he'd believed her to be a poor, deficient creature.

Now he realized how wrong he had been. Meriel's mind might be different from the minds of normal women, but she was not simple. She was as complex as he was, perhaps more so. Like a pagan nature spirit, she knew this land, these creatures, and had been willing to defend them no matter what the risk to herself. Now, because he had helped the fox, she was permitting him a glimpse into her soul.

She touched his hand briefly in an unmistakable sign of thanks. He wanted to capture that small, strong hand in his own so he could feel her warmth and strength. Instead he drew an unsteady breath. "I was glad to help, Meriel."

The awareness between them had been transformed. Any future relationship must be as equals.

Chapter 10

Even though he had become fully, unavoidably alive to her, she had not known he was a kindred spirit. Then with his words and touch and compassion he had ministered to the injured vixen. Even she had been unable to do that.

He had undeniable power. His healing work had brightened the golden energy that swirled around him. Slowly she rose to her feet. He did the same, his expression serious, gaze locked to hers. His eyes were a wondrous blue, alive with humor and intelligence. He looked not just *at* her, but *through* her.

She felt a quiver of alarm that someone might come so close, know so much. Yet like the vixen, her anxiety was tempered by instinctive trust.

She had thought there was not another being in the world anything like her.

Perhaps she was wrong.

After the incident with the fox, Dominic and Meriel returned to the house in companionable silence. Whatever imp had made her flee him earlier had vanished.

They ended up in the kitchen for an impromptu breakfast. Clearly Meriel's presence was commonplace, but having a viscount, even a fraudulent one, sent the cook and her assistants into spasms. It was one thing for a lord to order a picnic basket, quite another for him to sit down at a scrubbed pine table and enjoy eggs and toast and tea. He did his best to soothe them, but using Kyle's reserved manner made the task more difficult.

After they ate, Meriel headed out the back of the house to the parterre. Each of the raised flower beds was bordered by a low hedge of boxwood. Dominic had seen from the house how the hedges twined into elaborate patterns, with different sections separated by stone paths. From above the effect was beautifully geometric.

Today, several beds that had contained flowers past their prime had been cleared and prepared for new plantings. Handcarts full of sturdy plants waited on the paths. He realized that he was about to learn how much work was required to keep a formal garden beautiful.

Meriel marched to a cart and lifted the battered straw hat that someone, probably Kamal, had left for her. After setting it low on her head, she began removing flowers—pinks, he thought—from their nest of straw, and setting them on the raised, diamond-shaped bed. Each plant was precisely positioned equidistant from its fellows.

Taking a trowel from the cart, she knelt and moved the first pink to one side so she could dig a hole. When she was finished, she carefully lowered the flower into place and packed soil around it. Then she stood and handed Dominic the trowel, making a gesture that said quite plainly, "Show me if you can do this."

As he took the tool and knelt by the flower bed, he had the whimsical thought that she didn't talk because she didn't have to. When she wanted to make her wishes known, she could communicate very clearly indeed.

He dug with care, making sure that the hole was large enough to take the root ball without crowding. Then he set the plant inside and tamped earth firmly around the roots.

Feeling an absurd need for her approval, he glanced up at Meriel. Her face was shadowed by the wide brim of the shabby hat, but her nod indicated satisfaction. She moved to a different bed and began taking flowers from the adjacent cart.

Dominic grinned as he began to dig. Would the Earl of Wrexham be pleased to know that his disappointing younger son might be qualified for the job of undergardener? Whistling softly, he set the next pink into place.

As the sun moved to its zenith and slowly began to descend, Dominic learned that planting flowers was surprisingly satisfying. He'd zealously studied agriculture on the Dornleigh home farm. Wanting to understand everything, he had sowed seed, scythed hay, and harvested corn. The garden, though, had been his mother's particular charge, and he knew little about flowers other than the fact that he enjoyed them.

Now he discovered that working the soil with his bare hands was powerfully sensual. He liked the moist richness of the earth, the knowledge that his efforts would allow the frail, pretty blossoms to grow and flourish.

He thought of busy, frenetic London, where he would be if Kyle hadn't enlisted him for this charade. That world of fashionable activity and superficial relationships had been his life for years. Shropshire was very different. No wonder gardeners seemed so content. Kamal had a calm as wide as the whole outdoors.

Meriel in garden mode was also a restful companion. Occasionally he'd glance over to where she was working, and smile at the sight of her small bare feet. They were an endearing mixture of elegance and dirt, like the rest of her.

Not that he looked much more respectable. The morning's activities had fulfilled his vow to ruin one of Kyle's expensive coats. As the day warmed, he tossed the coat aside, rolled up the sleeves of his shirt, and generally looked like a perfect ragamuffin.

Completing a bed, he rose and stretched muscles and joints unaccustomed to planting. Then he crossed to Meriel so she could direct him to the bed she wanted done next. She wasn't working, though. For the first time in hours, she was simply sitting back on her heels, hands relaxed on her thighs.

Following her gaze, he saw that she was intently watching a yellow butterfly. Rather than interrupt, he settled beside her. He could scarcely see her features under the shadow of her absurd hat, but he was glad her delicate skin was protected from the midday sun. The fierce heat of India must have been cruel for someone of her coloring.

The minutes dragged by. What was so blasted interesting about a common yellow butterfly? The countryside was full of them. He began to study this one.

No question that butterflies were prettier than most insects. In fact, he'd never noticed how lovely the fragile golden wings looked with the light glowing through, emphasizing the tracery of darker veins. For such an insignificant creature, it was really quite complex. Interesting that the antennae were club shaped at the ends.

Having collected the nectar of one blossom, it drifted to another. He imagined himself flying like that, weightless and free. A pleasant fantasy, though it was easier to imagine Meriel as a butterfly, for she was a creature of lightness and grace.

Time slowed as he studied the butterfly and its leisurely progress around Meriel's flower bed. When it finally flew away, he blinked with surprise, wondering how long he'd been caught up in his observations. He hadn't watched an insect so closely since he was a small child, if then. Part of Meriel's special quality was her ability to become totally absorbed, like a child.

But now she was all business as she rose to her feet and ushered him to another bed and another cart of flowers. "You're a harsh taskmistress," he said teasingly as he took up his trowel again.

He was almost sure that he saw a wicked gleam in her eye before she turned away. Smiling, he started digging again.

About midafternoon, a pleasant, cultivated tenor voice said warmly, "Good day, Meriel. How are you?"

Startled because he hadn't heard footsteps, Dominic glanced up and saw a middle-aged gentleman of fair coloring and slight build crossing the parterre to where Meriel worked. She stood at his approach.

He kissed her lightly on the cheek. "My dear child. It's good to see you."

She tolerated the kiss, seeming neither pleased nor displeased. For an unguarded instant, the man's expression showed profound regret. Then he raised her work-hardened hands, regarding them ruefully. "I do wish you'd wear the gloves I gave you."

Warily Dominic got to his feet. Given the man's coloring, build, and expensive clothing, he was probably Meriel's uncle, Lord Amworth. But if Dominic guessed wrong, it would be a hard error to explain. Worse, Amworth knew Kyle better than anyone else at Warfield. He would be the most likely to see through the imposture.

The man glanced over when Dominic stood. His jaw dropped. "Lord Maxwell?"

In his brother's cool voice, Dominic said, "Have I managed to surprise you?"

"You have indeed." The newcomer's disbelieving gaze scanned the pretend Lord Maxwell. "I scarcely recognized you."

111

"It seemed advisable to enter into Lady Meriel's activities." Dominic allowed himself a faint smile. "She's quite willing to put me to work."

The man looked from Dominic to Meriel and back again. "Does she accept you in...in other ways?"

The man had to be Amworth, though Dominic resolved to avoid using the name until he had proof. "I've been moving slowly, so as not to alarm her."

"That's wise. Though as you know, time is not unlimited." His concerned gaze went to Meriel. "I was on my way to my own estate, and decided to come by and see how you were progressing."

"Will you stay the night?" Dominic asked, hoping the answer would be no.

He was out of luck. Amworth nodded. "I always enjoy visiting Warfield, especially at this season. Will you walk with me, Maxwell? I want to speak with you."

Desperate for an excuse to avoid a private conversation, Dominic said gravely, "I dare not abandon my task for fear my supervisor would become angry with me."

Amworth smiled a little. "Very well. Until later, then."

Gloomily Dominic watched the older man return to the house. He'd have to be on guard all evening. He hoped the ladies were in a talkative mood, since every time Dominic opened his mouth, he'd be in danger of putting his foot into it.

Dominic dressed with extra care that evening, even allowing Morrison to shave him. He was glad he'd made the effort when he saw that Amworth came down to dinner with full London formality. Mrs. Rector and Mrs. Marks were also dressed in their best.

After casual chat over sherry, he and Amworth escorted the ladies into the dining room. As always, a place was set for Meriel, though she hadn't dined with her chaperons since Dominic had arrived at Warfield.

Then Meriel appeared in the dining room doorway. Dominic looked up, and felt as if he'd been poleaxed. This was Meriel as he'd never seen her. Her shining hair was swept into a knot high on her head, revealing the slim elegance of her pearl-adorned neck. Her white gown glittered with silver embroidery, and when she stepped into the room he saw that she wore matching silver slippers.

Her appearance was so striking that it took him a moment to realize that the garment was at least thirty years out of date. Not that he cared—beautiful was beautiful. He almost fell over his own feet as he rose to escort her to the table. She wore perfume, a heady blend of spice and flowers.

"I'm so glad you're joining us, Meriel. We've missed you these last few days." Mrs. Rector glanced at Dominic. "Her mother's gown. Emily was also petite."

"Emily was something of a collector of exotic costumes, Lord Maxwell," Mrs. Marks

113

added. "Meriel has appeared in everything from Norwegian peasant dress to embroidered Chinese robes. No doubt she chose a more conventional garment in your honor, Lord Amworth."

Amworth rose, his gaze locked on his niece, pain in his eyes. "I remember this gown. Emily wore it the night she was presented. Meriel looks so much like her."

Dominic pulled back her chair. She sank into it as gracefully as drifting eiderdown, silken skirts whispering around her. Her gaze was cast down demurely like a girl from the schoolroom attending her first adult entertainment. Reminding himself of the minx who'd done her best to frighten him out of ten years of his life that morning, Dominic took his own seat again.

As the meal began, he pondered once more the question of how much Meriel understood. She recognized her uncle and apparently cared enough to dress to please him. Dominic liked the thought of her dressing up in her mother's clothes. His little sister had done the same when she was a child.

Though he'd only seen her eating with her fingers before, tonight she used knife and fork with perfect ease. She would have learned table manners as a child, before the tragedy that had disturbed her mind. Yet most of the time, she didn't choose to exercise the refinement she showed tonight.

He thought of the uncontrolled wildness she'd shown earlier when she attacked the poacher. Might she have—he groped for a concept—a personality made of disparate pieces? Wildness coexisting with docility? Danger lurking behind a dreamy facade?

He sighed. As usual, he had observations and questions, but no answers. Perhaps Lord Amworth could be induced to speak more of her condition over the port.

At the end of the meal, Mrs. Marks rose and gave the signal for the ladies to withdraw. Dominic would have to cope with Amworth on his own. The two men stood politely as the women left. Gazing after them, Dominic noticed that Meriel turned the opposite direction from the older women. He remarked as he took his seat again, "Meriel's conformity doesn't extend to sitting in the drawing room?"

"Not usually." Amworth reached for the port decanter that had been set out for the gentlemen. "Sometimes she'll join us later. I hope she does tonight. I don't see as much of her as I'd like." He poured for both of them, then settled back in his chair. "So tell me your thoughts now that you've had time to become better acquainted with my niece. Will she make you a wife?"

Dominic hesitated, wishing he could avoid this conversation. His distaste for the marriage of Meriel and Kyle grew greater with each hour. If he wanted to, he could spike the betrothal right now. But then what? Not only would he lose Bradshaw Manor, but Amworth might well turn to another prospective bridegroom. Kyle at least would not mistreat Meriel. She might do worse with another man.

"It's too soon to say," he temporized. "Meriel is a rare creature, in some ways a child, yet with her own kind of wisdom. I scarcely know what to make of her."

"My own thoughts exactly." Amworth leaned forward earnestly. "Surely the fact that you appreciate how special she is will make a good foundation for marriage."

"Perhaps from my point of view." Dominic hesitated. Then, knowing he'd hate himself if he didn't speak up, he continued, "But what about Meriel's needs? Might she not be happier if she is left alone? She seems content with her life."

"I wish it were that simple." Amworth sighed. "She needs a protector. Life is uncertain. If something were to happen to me, I fear for Meriel's welfare."

After a long silence, Dominic prompted, "What do you fear?"

The other man gave him a sharp glance. "We discussed this before, Maxwell."

Trying to cover his misstep, Dominic said smoothly, "I listened then without really knowing Meriel. I'd like to hear it all again now that my image of her is fuller."

Accepting that, Amworth said, "Her other uncle, Lord Grahame, has thought from the beginning that she might do better in an asylum. Several times he has sent doctors who specialize in madness to examine her, and all have agreed."

Dominic's brows arched. "They think she can be successfully treated?"

Amworth's mouth twisted. "Oh, no one suggested there was any chance she would ever be normal. But doctors are curious brutes. I think they liked the idea of experimenting to see what might help." He stared down into his port. "Perhaps she would improve at a modern asylum and my stubbornness is selfish. But I...I can't bear to think of her locked away in such a place. I've kept news of her occasional bad spells away from Grahame for fear he'd use them as evidence to remove her from Warfield."

The thought of Meriel subjected to medical experiments made Dominic shudder. "If that's selfishness, I'm selfish, too. I can't imagine her anywhere but here."

Amworth looked up, his gaze intense. "One of the reasons I want you for Meriel's husband is that you have the reputation of being a man of honor. If you marry her, promise me that you'll never lock her away."

Dominic looked down at his port as he thought how the honorable Kyle had sent a substitute in his place. "There is no marriage yet."

"There won't be one unless you promise that she stays here, where she is happy, and that she is cared for with kindness and dignity," Amworth said harshly.

Choosing his words, Dominic said, "I swear that no matter what happens, whether I marry her or not, I shall always protect her to the best of my abilities." And if Kyle would not swear a similar vow, Dominic would tell Amworth the truth of this deception.

The older man gave a sigh of relief. Rising to his feet, he said, "Before we rejoin the ladies, would you care for a stroll through the gallery upstairs?"

Knowing the suggestion wasn't casual, Dominic said, "Of course."

Silently he accompanied Amworth to the gallery, a long room on the north side of the house. A gentle promenade in bad weather, it had wide, diamond-paned windows on one wall and paintings on the other. Amworth stopped at a portrait near the entrance and lifted his lamp so light fell clearly across the canvas.

The picture portrayed a smiling young woman with flaxen hair sitting on a stone garden bench. On her lap was a small and angelically lovely little girl with sparkling light green eyes, while a craggy man with humor and intelligence in his gaze stood behind. If Dominic wasn't mistaken, the setting was the Warfield rose garden. "Your sister and her husband with Meriel, I assume."

"It was done just before they went to India." Amworth gazed broodingly at the painting. "They had been married for years and had begun to despair of having a child. Then Meriel came. They both doted on her."

"Why did Lord Grahame take his family to an unhealthy place like India?"

"Emily wouldn't hear of him going without her, and she wouldn't go without Meriel. Grahame's mission was for only two years, so they thought it would be safe enough. Meriel was a remarkably healthy child." He closed his eyes for a moment, his expression bleak. "It wasn't disease that killed my sister and her husband."

"You and your sister were very close?"

Amworth's eyes opened. His face looked very worn. "Emily was only a year younger. We were constant companions as children, and stayed friends until she died."

The property ownership question intrigued Dominic. Grahame and Amworth both had family seats, while Emily had owned Warfield in her own right, and apparently she and her husband had used it as their primary residence. He'd better not ask about that, though; it might be something else Amworth and Kyle had discussed.

They walked along the bank of paintings. Many of the portraits showed men and women who were small-boned and very blond. The women often had Meriel's fey, otherworldly air. Dominic remarked, "The family resemblance is very marked."

Amworth stopped by a Tudor family portrait. "I wish there was a picture of the first Meriel. The family archives indicate that she was much like my niece, except that she had black hair. Her husband, a Norman earl, was very blond. Those traits have come down through the family for centuries. Family names and titles have changed, but the blood has carried on, often through female inheritance. Warfield was never made part of an entail, so it could be left to a daughter if there was no male heir. My niece is a direct descendant of the first Meriel." He sighed. "I hate to think that will all end now."

"Surely there are other branches of the family."

"True. But my own sons look more like their mother." He hesitated before adding with some difficulty, "Elinor has been an ideal wife and mother and countess, but...she has never been able to accept Meriel. She finds mental imbalance disturbing. When the boys were small she was concerned for their safety."

He didn't need to say any more. Dominic understood how Amworth had been torn between the demands of his position, the needs of his own family, and those of his niece. Probably he would have taken her into his own household if his wife had not objected. He'd done the best he could to see that Meriel was loved and happy.

He and his niece both deserved better than a pair of liars.

Chapter 11

After a pleasant evening of conversation, a tea tray was delivered to the drawing room. Mrs. Marks was pouring for Lord Amworth when Meriel materialized in the doorway. She'd changed from her evening gown into a flowing dark Eastern garment, the kind designed to cover as much as possible of the female form to prevent lustful male thoughts. Not that it worked. The folds of dark fabric merely stimulated the imagination. At least they stimulated Dominic's.

Carrying a tray with three small bowls and a cluster of slender sticks, Meriel crossed the Persian carpet on soundless bare feet. Her hair had been released from its complicated style and braided again. Mrs. Rector smiled. "How nice. Meriel is going to do mehndi tonight in your honor, Lord Amworth."

Eyes downcast, Meriel knelt before her uncle. Dominic had a sudden sense that the role of submissive handmaiden was a game for her. Perhaps she'd seen the real thing in India and added it to the collection of her personalities. Submissive Handmaiden. Dedicated Gardener. Fairy Sprite. Wild Child.

Amworth's tired face lightened. "I'd like a wrist band if you please, Meriel." He rolled his left sleeve up and offered her his wrist.

She dunked a pad of cotton into a bowl and sponged the skin around his wrist. Then she dipped a slim stick into the other bowl, which contained henna paste. With swift, deft motions, she began to draw a complex, paisleylike pattern on his wrist. Her concentration was total. As Dominic had thought after seeing the mehndi on Kamal, it took skill to create such a design, particularly without guidelines.

He noted with interest that she'd darkened her brows and lashes, as Eastern women often did. Against Meriel's fair skin and flaxen

121

hair, the effect was exotic and wickedly alluring.

When she'd finished Amworth's mehndi, she went to Mrs. Rector. The older woman said thoughtfully, "I'd like an anklet, Meriel. Will you gentlemen excuse me while I turn my back on you for modesty's sake?"

She moved to a large wing chair that faced away from the fireplace, where the others were seated. Fabric rustled as she raised her skirts and peeled off a stocking so Meriel could work on her ankle. Dominic sipped his tea, amused and rather touched at this evidence that a woman didn't lose the playful desire to adorn herself merely because she was no longer a girl.

The anklet took some time to execute. When it was completed, Mrs. Marks proffered her right hand and arm. Meriel drew a delicate vinelike pattern that started on the older woman's third finger. From there the mehndi wound across the back of Mrs. Marks's hand and wrist, continuing up her forearm before it twined to a halt just below the elbow.

As Meriel worked, Mrs. Marks explained, "It's necessary to leave the henna on for an hour or two until it dries, Lord Maxwell. Then it can be brushed off, leaving the pattern." Her eyes twinkled. "I suppose this seems very odd to you."

"Unusual," he admitted, "but quite charming."

He was looking forward to Meriel's ministrations, but after she finished with Mrs. Marks, she made the rounds of her three subjects and patted a solution from the third bowl on the designs, then gracefully withdrew. Disappointed, he wondered if she had run out of the henna preparation. Or wasn't he worthy of her efforts?

Mrs. Rector got to her feet, covering a ladylike yawn with one small hand. "It is rather late, isn't it? I shall see you all in the morning."

Since Meriel was gone, Dominic was ready to retire. Was it really only this morning that he'd followed her up to the castle? Much had happened in one day.

Morrison awaited in the bedroom to help him out of Kyle's fashionably tight coat. The valet would not soon forgive Dominic for wrecking the garment he'd worn earlier in the day. Not in the mood for the older man's disapproval, Dominic dismissed him after the coat was off. The rest of his clothing he could manage unaided.

Glad to be alone, Dominic wandered to the window as he unfastened his cravat. Outside, the geometric patterns of the parterre were faintly visible in the moonlight. He'd always enjoyed this view, never more than now, when he'd labored on it himself.

His door opened and he turned, thinking Morrison had forgotten something.

Meriel stood in the doorway, dressed in her Eastern costume and holding her mehndi tray. Closing the door behind her, she crossed the room to Dominic and knelt demurely at his feet, fluid garments swirling. Then she raised the tray in a wordless offer.

He cut off his automatic protest that young ladies never came to gentlemen's bedrooms. Meriel existed outside society's usual rules. "So my turn has come." He smiled at her. "Will you give me a wristband like your uncle's?"

She gestured toward the upholstered chair. He sat and unbuttoned his cuff so she could paint his wrist, glad he hadn't been excluded from her list of subjects.

Taking his hand with smooth, cool fingers, she studied his wrist with a frown.

"Is something wrong?" He looked down and guessed that the hair on his wrist might interfere with her painting. He was about to suggest that Meriel put a design on the back of his hand when she stood and quite unself-consciously began unfastening his shirt buttons. He caught her hand, startled. "Meriel!"

She raised her head and looked at him with such transparent innocence that he felt ashamed of himself. Now that he thought about it, Kamal had mehndi on the throat, so this was probably a standard practice for her.

Reminding himself that it was a good thing for her to become comfortable with a man's body, he finished undoing his shirt and pulled it over his head. Though he felt some embarrassment at being half-naked in front of her, Meriel was quite unconcerned. She perched on the arm of the chair and thoughtfully traced his collarbone with a fingertip, apparently considering her design.

His blood began beating with uncomfortable force, for her light touch was more arousing than a caress from a practiced woman of the world. Kamal had the advantage of being a eunuch, and her sworn protector. Safe from the provocative lure of a maiden's touch. Dominic had no such defenses.

Decision made, Meriel cleansed his skin with a fluid whose tangy scent reminded him of pine. Then she dipped a stick into the henna and began to draw on the triangle of flesh above his left collarbone. As the rich, earthy scent filled his nostrils, he had a charming view of her bright hair and the occasional sweep of darkened lashes.

Too charming. He closed his eyes and tried to fasten his mind on other things—Latin declensions were suitably tedious—but his attention came stubbornly back to her. Blending with the other scents was a tantalizing perfume, and he could feel the warmth radiating from her hand. The drawing stick produced a sensation somewhere between a tickle and a sensual tease, and why hadn't he noticed how warm the room was...?

He opened his eyes again and stared across the room at the Chinese wallpaper. Forget that an exquisite young woman was hovering over him. Pretend she was some incredibly gnarled old hag he'd discovered in a bazaar in Damascus....

She lifted the stick from his skin, and he heard a faint tap as she rested it in the bowl. Then her fingertip rubbed across his nipple. He almost jumped from his skin. "Jesus, Meriel!"

She looked at him with that innocence

again. "This is really not at all proper, Meriel," he said unsteadily. "You should return to your room."

Ignoring that, she prepared his skin, then drew a delicate, vinelike design around his nipple. Did she do this to Kamal? Even if she did, should he allow such intimacy?

What the devil should he do? He didn't want to distress her—but damn it, she was distressing *him*! All he could think about was her nearness, and her desirability. He could almost taste the soft skin of her nape under his lips....

Grimly he held on to his fraying willpower while she painted a design around his other nipple, then decorated the area above his right collarbone. With a final flourish, she connected the two areas with a web of lines that curved across the base of his throat.

He gave a sigh of relief when she finished and set her materials on the table beside the chair. Now she would go back to her room, and he would read something quietly while the henna dried. He could surely find some deadly dull improving work in the library to cool himself off.

But instead of moving away, she slid her hand caressingly down his chest in a slow, sensual exploration. Fire shot through his veins as the desire that had been building kindled into flame. He almost reached up to pull her into a crushing embrace.

Almost. With barely suppressed violence he shoved himself from the chair and didn't stop until he was on the far side of the room. Back turned to her, he clenched his hands, breathing hard as he fought to maintain his control.

She was fey. At least half mad. Not responsible for her actions. *She was going to be his brother's wife.*

Would she even notice the difference between him and Kyle on their wedding night? The bitterness of that thought dampened his craving.

He turned and found that she was right beside him, a question in her eyes. She lifted a hand toward him. He caught it before she could touch him again. "Meriel, this kind of closeness is only proper between husband and wife. Until you are ready to be a wife, there should be...more distance between us."

He hoped that she understood the tone if not the words, but she just stared at him, her green eyes intense. Not the eyes of a child at all.

Her gaze dropped, sliding over his body with slow thoroughness as if she was memorizing every pore, every hair, every taut muscle. Feeling profoundly naked under that probing gaze, he ordered, "Go, Meriel. *Now.*"

Her gaze reached the front of his pantaloons. He hardened as if she'd touched him physically. He knew with absolute certainty that he could draw her into a kiss, and she would come willingly. She was curious. Naturally sensual. She probably wore nothing underneath that flowing, exotic garment....

His brother's wife. He turned her around, placed a tense hand in the small of her back, and ushered her firmly to the door. "Begone, witch. No more mehndi until your wedding night."

Kyle would have to be dead not to become an ardent bridegroom under the influence of Meriel's enchanting blend of innocence and sensuality. His thrice-damned brother, who still commanded Dominic's loyalty even though he might not deserve it.

He closed the door hard behind her and turned the key in the lock.

Then he leaned against the Chinese wallpaper, and shook.

She almost fell over Roxana, who thumped her tail happily at the sight of Meriel. Feeling like a bird whose feathers had been ruffled by a high wind, she stood very still and tried to understand what had just happened.

He really was quite beautiful. She'd enjoyed the feel of smooth, taut skin that was several shades darker than her own. The texture and elegant patterning of the hair that dusted across his chest and arrowed downward so intriguingly. As she drew the mehndi, his energy had come alive, swirling into the crimson of desire. She had wanted to touch him all over, taste him and let him taste her....

Furiously impatient, she whirled and marched down the corridor to the back stairs, her private entry and exit. For once she shut Roxana indoors, preferring to be alone. Every sensation was magnified as she stalked through the cool night air. Scents floated seductively on the breeze, the dew-touched grass was cool beneath her feet. She felt painfully restless and alive.

Moving soundlessly through alternating patches of moonlight and shadows, she entered the wilderness area. The illusion of untamed forest suited her mood. An owl hooted as it passed above her so closely she heard the beat of wings. A moment later, a death shriek revealed that the hunter had found prey.

A deeper scream, drawn out and eerie, cut through the woods. A badger, she thought, though more often they growled or barked. Curious, she followed the sound.

A hundred paces farther she came to the edge of a small clearing where a pair of badgers leaped and tumbled in a mating dance. The female reared onto her hind legs, her masked face dramatic in the moonlight. Looking like a waltz partner, the male did the same, eager to charm and impress her. They came together and rolled over the soft turf in a patchwork furry ball.

All coy teasing, the female darted in to snap at the male's shoulder. He reared up, then roughly pinned her down, biting at her neck before starting to lick her dark fur with possessive tenderness. The female made a low, almost catlike purring sound as she quivered with anticipation.

Their intoxicated play was the warp and weft of a species' survival, a passionate attraction so intense they did not even notice her presence. Blindly Meriel turned away, her mind vivid with images. Tumbling rapturously with Renbourne in a meadow. Her teeth nipping his warm, hard body as play turned to passion. His mouth, his hands, teasing her to wildness, his strength vanquishing hers as he possessed her willing body.

She was in the moon garden before her sensual haze dissipated enough for her to notice her surroundings. The intoxicating fragrance of mock orange hung heavy in the air, and around her beds of white flowers showed ghostly pale in the moonlight. In the center of the garden, trailing blossoms spilled lushly from an ancient Roman urn. She dropped, shivering, onto the cool stone dais supporting the sculpture.

All creatures mated. She'd known that, had observed most of the birds and beasts of Warfield in their swift passions. The female went into heat, and the male went mad with yearning. The behavior was intriguing, and she'd learned how male and female bodies came together, but she'd never understood the urge. Indeed, she'd been grateful to be spared such wildness.

Now she realized that she had been spared only because she had not met her true mate. For the first time she comprehended that fierce craving to join with another. Secret places in her body pulsed with hunger even though she knew instinctively that tonight she had tasted only the merest sip of passion's cup. There was more, so much more.

But humankind, in its foolishness, made

everything so difficult. Renbourne wanted her. She had seen desire in his eyes, scented it on his body, seen the bright blaze of his energy when she touched him.

Yet he had held back for some barbaric, unnatural reason. A nuisance, that. But he was male, and young, and his blood beat hot and wild in his veins. Her time would come. She knew it in her bones.

He was her true mate, and soon he would be hers.

Chapter 12

Staying awake while the mehndi dried was easy; getting to sleep at all was the problem. Dominic eventually fell into a restless slumber, and a vivid dream of making love to Meriel. He awoke to an empty bed with his heart hammering and the knowledge that his body had entered into his dream with embarrassing thoroughness.

After washing his face, he brushed off the dried henna. The mehndi resembled a paisley collar composed of light orange lines. There was a barbaric, un-English splendor to seeing his skin patterned.

He turned from the mirror abruptly when he thought of her small, skilled hands moving over him. After the last night, it was impossible to deny how powerfully he was attracted to her. Very well, he was attracted. What man wouldn't be? What mattered was controlling his inappropriate desire.

The morning did not improve when he went down to breakfast and learned that Lord Amworth was already gone. Feeling ill-bred for not having risen in time to take leave of the older man, Dominic poured a cup of coffee in the hope it would restore him.

He was working on his second cup when Mrs. Rector drifted into the breakfast parlor and poured herself some tea. As she settled at the table, she remarked, "Lord Amworth was pleased that you and Meriel are getting along so well."

Deciding some mature insight might be helpful, he said, "I value her, but I'm not sure about the wisdom of marriage. What have the physicians who examined her said?"

Mrs. Rector pursed her lips. "Nothing consistent. They all agreed she was not normal—as if one needed to study in Edinburgh to see that!—and they agreed on nothing else. Most thought she would benefit by intensive treatment in an asylum, but they all had their pet ideas about what sort of treatment might work."

That wasn't a great deal of help. "Are any of those physicians in this area?"

"Dr. Craythorne is one of the foremost authorities on madness in England. He has an asylum at Bladenham, only ten miles away." A touch of irony entered her voice. "It's said to be very progressive."

"Do you believe Meriel would benefit by a course of treatment?"

She gazed out the window without seeing. "If I believed that, I'd have taken her to Bladenham myself. But then, I'm a second cousin of Meriel's mother. Fey females run in the family." She smiled wryly. "I'm not so very practical myself."

He thought about what she was saying. "You feel that Meriel is more of an...an intensification of the family type than she is a true madwoman?"

Mrs. Rector nodded. "How can a physician cure what's bred in the bone?"

She might have a point, but Dominic would still like to hear the doctor's opinion. In fact, now that he thought about it, the idea of getting away from Warfield and Meriel for the day was very, very appealing.

"Lord Maxwell, what a pleasure!" Dr. Craythorne, tall, solid, and inspiring confidence, strode across the handsomely appointed reception room where Dominic had been brought by the porter.

So far, Bladenham was impressive. A sprawling house on the edge of a village, it was spacious and well furnished, with a large walled garden at the back. Not a hellhole at all.

"How may I help you?" the doctor continued.

Dominic was beginning to appreciate why

Kyle was so fond of being the heir; nothing like a title to get instant deference. "I understand that you have examined Lady Meriel Grahame. I am interested in your conclusions."

Craythorne hesitated. "Such discussion is usually limited to a patient's family."

"Which I might become," Dominic said dryly. "Do you take my meaning?"

The doctor did. Shaking his head, he said, "Such a sad case. Her paternal uncle, Lord Grahame, appreciates the benefits of modern treatment, but her other guardian has been obdurate. He simply refuses to see reason. It's almost as if he doesn't wish her...." He cut himself off. "Forgive me for saying that. Lord Amworth surely desires the best for his niece, but his attitude has been hopelessly old-fashioned."

"I'm aware of the disagreement between her ladyship's uncles," Dominic said in a neutral voice. "Since a marriage is being considered, I feel I should know as much as possible about her condition."

Craythorne's expression brightened as he realized that a husband would have jurisdiction over his wife's treatment, and could overrule an obstructive uncle. "I've examined the girl several times over the years, and I can say with absolute certainty that allowing her to run wild is the worst possible treatment. Regular habits are essential to establishing self-control. Without such discipline, her behavior has worsened."

Dominic frowned. "In what way?"

"She grows increasingly irrational. The

last time I paid a call, she led me up to the old castle, then staged a suicide attempt. I feared for her life." His face darkened. "I was on the verge of sending riverboats to search for her body when she reappeared, looking bland as butter."

Dominic almost laughed. So he wasn't the only one the little witch had played that trick on! But how could the doctor think her undisciplined after seeing her gardens? Keeping his expression grave, he said, "What type of treatment would you use with her?"

"First and most important, she should be removed from whatever pernicious influences affect her at Warfield. We would immediately establish a structured routine for her. After that, it would vary. I employ a range of therapies, depending on how the patient responds." Craythorne's heavy brows drew together. "Let me take you on a tour of our facilities. That will answer your questions better than mere words."

Glad the doctor had anticipated his request, Dominic followed the other man from the office into a corridor that ran toward the west wing of the house. It stopped at a massive, iron-bound door. Craythorne opened it with a large key from a jangling ring.

Fashionable furnishings vanished on the other side of the door. The corridor was starkly whitewashed, without decoration of any kind. "It's important not to overstimulate the patients," the doctor explained. "Most have far too much going on in their brains already, overheating their blood and imbalancing the humors."

They walked down the dim, echoing corridor. Despite impeccable cleanliness, a faint miasma of uncontrolled bodily functions permeated the air.

Craythorne stopped by a door and indicated a small covered window for viewing inside. "Patients must learn self-control. This is one of two restraint rooms."

Dominic lifted the hinged cover and peered inside. The room was immaculately clean but utterly austere. A wooden chair was bolted to the floor, and a burly man in a straitjacket was tied to it. His head hung in an image of despair that chilled Dominic's blood. "Are patients routinely tied up here?"

"Mr. Enoch is one of our most difficult cases, and has spent a great deal of time in restraints. I believe, however, that he is beginning to understand that bad behavior is punished, while good behavior is rewarded. A salutary fear is a great aid to encouraging self-discipline. As his understanding improves, restraints will be needed less and less."

Dominic thought of Meriel tied to a chair like that one, and his stomach turned over. "Is such treatment suitable for a delicate female?"

"Narcotics and tonics are usually effective in soothing agitated females, but occasionally the restraints are required," the doctor said with regret. "But unlike most asylums, I will not allow patients to be put in chains, no matter how severe the case."

Dominic supposed that was a sign of enlightenment. If Bladenham was progressive, what in the name of heaven were other asylums like?

Craythorne resumed walking along the corridor. "Down at the end we have the ice bath room. Ice is shipped down from Scotland every winter to ensure an adequate supply. It is not an insignificant cost, but I assure you, Lord Maxwell, we spare no expense when it comes to patient treatment."

A resounding crash shattered the silence, followed by a bellow of obscenities. Swearing under his breath, Craythorne quickened his pace. "Mr. Jones is having one of his spells. When you see him, you will understand the need for restraints."

Three large men dressed in gray came racing toward them from the other end of the hall. Their chief unlocked Mr. Jones's room, and they rushed inside.

Curious, Dominic wanted to follow, too, but Craythorne blocked him with an outstretched arm. "Don't," he said tersely. "It's not safe."

Looking through the open door, Dominic saw a room so plain, it was more cell than bedchamber. The only furniture was a cot that had apparently been bolted to the floor. Mr. Jones, a surprisingly small man, had ripped the cot loose and was wielding it like a weapon as he shouted filthy words in a hoarse voice. He swung wildly at his keepers. Two of the attendants managed to dodge him, but the other was trapped against a wall. The cot smashed into his ribs, and he collapsed with a cry of pain.

Before Jones could swing the cot again, the other two attendants tackled him to the floor. Even with the advantage of size and number, they could barely hold the frenzied patient down.

During the struggle that followed, Craythorne slipped away for a moment, then returned with a coarse canvas straitjacket. With the skill of practice, the attendants forced the garment over the patient's head and immobilized his arms. That done, the chief keeper shoved a handkerchief in Jones's mouth, cutting off the ugly words. A gag was tied over the man's mouth, and he was hauled to his feet.

As Jones was taken away, Craythorne explained, "He's going to the other restraint room. I'd thought the course of ice baths was helping him, but this is a serious relapse."

The attendant who'd been struck by the cot limped from the cell, pain in his face. "I think 'e cracked my ribs, sir."

"That was quite a blow you took," Craythorne said with concern. "Go to the infirmary. I'll examine you when I've finished showing Lord Maxwell around."

Sickened by the sight of such uncontrolled lunacy, Dominic fell in beside the doctor as they retraced their steps through the main block of the house. As Craythorne unlocked another door, he said, "Male patients are kept in the west wing, females in the east. They are always strictly segregated, and cared for by attendants of their own gender. Bladenham

138

has never had the kind of revolting scandal that some asylums have experienced."

It took a moment for Dominic to realize that the doctor was alluding to several notorious cases where female lunatics had been ravished and impregnated by male patients. And worse, sometimes the assailants had been keepers. Dear God, to think that afflicted women like Meriel were subjected to such savage treatment!

The first cell Dominic checked was empty, but sounds of hopeless sorrow came from the next. He looked in the peephole. A disheveled woman crouched in one corner of the cell, her arms wrapped around her knees as she rocked back and forth. Her sobbing would make angels weep.

Face rigid, he closed the hinged window plate. "What is her story?"

"Mrs. Wicker had more than a dozen miscarriages," the doctor said with compassion. "Only the first child was brought to term, and it died almost immediately. Last year, she descended into uncontrollable madness."

Dominic couldn't blame her. What kind of husband would subject his wife to such a series of disastrous pregnancies? "How are you treating her?"

"Leeches applied to the temples to draw off the evil humors have been the most effective," Craythorne said. "Along with purging and weekly bloodletting. She hasn't had a violent spell in weeks."

Ice baths. Straitjackets. Leeches and purging.

No wonder Amworth refused to consider sending Meriel here. Even if a cure was guaranteed, Dominic didn't think he could subject her to such treatment. As the grim tour continued, he asked, "Do many patients become well enough to return to their normal lives?"

"Some." The doctor's expression turned bleak. "I've had the best success with females suffering from melancholic complaints. In time, I believe that medicine will be able to cure all mental illness, but I don't expect it to happen in my lifetime."

At least Craythorne was honest, but Dominic wouldn't want Meriel in his care. She wasn't melancholic—she was sunshine personified. Or sometimes like a swift squall, but never melancholic. "Are patients confined to their rooms at all times?"

"Walking in the garden is one of the privileges extended for good behavior. Let me take you there."

Outdoor exercise sounded refreshing compared to the bleak misery of the rest of Bladenham. The garden was something of a disappointment, however. It consisted mostly of graveled paths and patches of lawn, with a few scattered shrubs and benches. Perhaps flower beds were considered overstimulating.

The high stone walls were topped with inward curving spikes. If this was the most progressive mental asylum in Britain, Dominic quite sincerely hoped he would die rather than ever be struck by madness.

Seeing the direction of Dominic's glance, the doctor said, "We've never had a patient escape. The village considers us the best of neighbors."

On the far side of the garden, two burly, gray-clad women followed several steps behind a pair of female patients. As the group turned and headed toward the house, Dominic saw how the older woman, on the left, stared vacantly past him. Her watery gaze had a terrifying blankness.

The other patient looked directly at Dominic, and he saw something swift and intense flicker in her eyes. A tall young woman with strong features and ragged dark hair, she might have been handsome under other circumstances.

Craythorne said in a low voice, "The woman on the left, Mrs. Gill, may be going home soon. She was suicidal, but is now quite calm. Mineral tonics and narcotic potions have soothed her agitation."

Soothed the poor woman into near unconsciousness, from what Dominic could see. "And the other patient?"

"Mrs. M— " He broke off without completing the name. "That patient is known as Mrs. Brown. Though her husband wishes the best care for her, he fears his neighbors learning of her condition. I believe he has told them that she is in Italy, for her lungs, while she is treated here. A pity that he feels he must spin a web of lies."

Her husband was not alone in his attitude; Dominic knew other families who denied cases of madness in their midst. "Is she improving?"

"She'll have long lucid spells, then go completely mad, particularly when her husband visits. I've had to ask him to come less often. I wish I could offer the poor devil more hope, but her behavior is so unpredictable that I cannot be sanguine." Craythorne regarded the patients, expression brooding. "If you'll excuse me a moment." With a nod, he went to speak to one of the attendants.

Dominic strolled toward a wall, thinking how poor a place this was compared to Meriel's vibrant, imaginative gardens. Then a shout echoed through the enclosure. He turned to see that Mrs. "Brown" had bolted and was running wild-eyed toward Dominic, her attendants pounding after her with all their might.

Dominic hadn't feared a woman since he left the nursery, but might a strong, healthy lunatic be a threat? Still, he'd be damned if he'd run from a female. He braced himself. But Mrs. Brown didn't attack. Instead she caught his arm, saying desperately, "Please, sir, I'm not mad! I'm being held here for no reason. If you'll take word to my father, he'll see I'm released. General Ames of Holliwell Grange. Please, I beg of you...."

Before she could say more, her keepers had caught up. Mrs. Brown dropped to her knees and wrapped her arms around Dominic's legs. "Ames of Holliwell Grange! In the name of God, just a note, anything to let him know so he can come for me!"

The attendants wrenched her away from Dominic as Dr. Craythorne arrived. "Your father knows you're here, Mrs. Brown, but he is too distressed by your condition to visit," he said in a gently implacable voice. "You know that—your husband has explained it to you over and over."

"My husband is a *liar!*" Her wild gaze went to Dominic again. "It was my husband who brought me here, and do you know why? Because I wasn't a biddable wife. Because my blood was impure. *Because I didn't agree with him!*"

Before she could say more, one keeper gagged her while the other wrestled her arms behind her back, dragging them up painfully. The attendants took Mrs. Brown away, leaving Dominic shaken.

"I think it is vital to always be honest with patients, but she is still prey to delusions as well as fits of violence," Craythorne said quietly. "I've seen no signs of progress. Luckily her husband can afford to keep her here with the best possible care. Perhaps, God willing, someday..." His voice faded away.

Knowing he would remember Mrs. Brown's frantic eyes until the day he died, Dominic turned and followed Craythorne into the house. He didn't doubt that the doctor was sincere and capable, and he ran his asylum well. But Dominic made a solemn oath that he would never let Meriel be sent to a place like this.

Chapter 13

Unable to shake his dark mood even after he left the asylum, Dominic rode back to Warfield more slowly than he'd taken the outward trip to Bladenham. Though vowing to protect Meriel from confinement was all very well, it was Kyle who would have authority over her person. Any decisions would be his.

He reminded himself that his brother could be an arrogant bastard, but he was never cruel to women. Even if Meriel descended into hopeless madness, surely he would keep her safely at Warfield, where she could enjoy fresh air and flowers and kindness.

But if he didn't, what would Dominic be able to do about it?

Arriving at the intersection of several roads, he glanced up at the half-dozen signs on the fingerpost. One said Holliwell.

"Take word to my father...General Ames of Holliwell Grange. Please, I beg of you...." A shiver went down Dominic's spine even though he told himself that a nearby Holliwell meant nothing, for the name was not uncommon. Mrs. Brown was mad, and nothing she said could be trusted. And yet....

He turned Pegasus toward Holliwell. He'd ride into the village and find that there was no Grange, and no General Ames. Then he could return to Warfield with a clear conscience. Losing an hour was a small price to pay for banishing those frantic dark eyes.

Within minutes, Dominic came abreast of a massive pair of stone gateposts. "Holliwell" was carved on the left post, and "Grange" on the right. He reined in his mount with a frown. This still proved nothing because every village in England had at least one house called a grange. Perhaps in better days Mrs. Brown had visited here.

But Holliwell Grange might really be owned by a General Ames who was her father, and who was so distressed by his daughter's madness that he couldn't bear to visit her. An inquiry from Dominic might do nothing more than bring further sorrow to a grieving parent. He steeled himself for that, since he would not forgive himself if he turned back when he was so close to learning the truth.

A few minutes' ride up a pleasant drive brought the grange into view. As the name implied, the building had started life as a farmhouse, but additions over the years had produced a large, rambling stone structure. Though not elegant, it looked comfortable and spacious, and prosperous fields and pastures lay in all directions.

Like many old farmsteads, the house comprised one side of a courtyard formed by outbuildings and a paddock. Dominic rode into the yard to tether his horse before trying the door. As he entered, a gentleman in country buckskins led a small, silvery gray mare from the stables.

"What a beauty!" Dominic said involuntarily.

The man glanced up. Tall and grizzled and ramrod straight, he could easily be a retired general. "Moonbeam is as well behaved as she is pretty." His admiring gaze went over Pegasus. "I see that you've a good eye for horseflesh."

"I like to think so, but what man doesn't?" Dominic firmly restrained Pegasus, who showed signs of wanting to pursue too close an acquaintance with the mare.

The older man turned Moonbeam into the paddock. After closing the gate, he turned to his visitor. His skin was dark and leathery, as if exposed to years of harsh sun. "I'm Ames, if you're looking for me."

For a moment Dominic froze, caught between names. Reminding himself that he couldn't be Dominic so close to Warfield, he dismounted from his horse. "My name is Maxwell. I'm staying at Warfield."

"Then you must know little Lady Meriel," Ames said with interest. "How is the child doing?"

"She's not a child anymore." Dominic tethered Pegasus, then joined Ames at the railing of the paddock. They contemplated the mare in respectful silence, bound together by the camaraderie of horsemen. Willing to postpone the purpose of his visit a little longer, Dominic added, "Lady Meriel is twenty-three now. You've met her?"

Ames pursed his lips in a soundless whistle. "How time passes. I haven't seen the girl since she was a child in India, but our families have been Shropshire neighbors for centuries. I thought of calling on her when I returned from the East several years ago, but given the stories of her mental state, I thought it better not to risk reminding the girl of what happened there." He shook his head. "Such a tragedy. I've always wondered if I could have done something to prevent her parents' deaths."

Dominic fitted that information with what he already knew. "You look like a military man. Were you stationed in India when Lord and Lady Grahame were killed?"

Ames nodded soberly. "Grahame was on a parliamentary mission that took him all over India. I commanded the army cantonment in Cambay, in the north. It was the last British outpost the Grahames visited before they were killed. From Cambay they traveled to Alwari, a minor residence of one of the local rulers. That's where the raiders struck. The whole palace was burned down, and a hundred people or so died." He sighed. "Very hard on Grahame's brother—the present Lord Grahame, that is."

"He was traveling with the party?" Dominic asked, wondering how the younger Grahame had survived the massacre.

The general shook his head. "No, he was a major serving under my command. A good officer—spoke Urdu like a native. The late Lord Grahame included Cambay on his route partly to visit his brother, because they hadn't seen each other in years. After the massacre Major

Grahame was distraught, of course. Kept saying that if his brother hadn't come to Cambay, he wouldn't have died."

"At least Lady Meriel survived. That must be some comfort."

Ames's expression eased. "She was the most intrepid little thing. She had a little gray pony, and she would tear across the plains like an Afghan bandit. Most mothers would have fainted on the spot, but Lady Grahame just laughed and urged her on."

"Lady Meriel could ride?" Dominic asked, startled.

"Since the age of three, according to her parents."

But not since. No wonder she had enjoyed riding with Dominic once she got over her initial anxiety. The experience must have brought back the happier days of her childhood. On impulse, he asked, "Is Moonbeam for sale? She looks like a perfect ladies' mount. I'd like to give her to Lady Meriel."

"I'd not thought of selling her. But for Lady Meriel?" Ames's eyes became distant. "Whenever I think of the girl, I also think of my daughter. Jena was several years older, so she appointed herself Meriel's guide and took her all over the encampment while the Grahames were at Cambay. The men adored them both."

Dominic's pulse quickened. "You have a daughter?"

"I did," Ames said curtly. Perhaps thinking that was too abrupt, he added with difficulty, "She died the autumn before last."

Ames seemed to be telling the truth, but it was possible that he preferred to tell others that his daughter was dead rather than admit to the shame of a mad child. Watching the older man closely, Dominic said, "I've just come from visiting the Bladenham asylum. While I was there, a patient begged me to take a message to her father, General Ames of Holliwell Grange. She said that she was not mad, that her husband had committed her to the asylum against her will."

The older man went bone white under his weathered skin, his pain palpable. "That's not possible. My daughter is dead."

Acutely uncomfortable, Dominic said, "I'm sorry. Probably the woman is someone from the neighborhood who knows Holliwell Grange, and in her madness thinks that she once lived here. I'm very sorry to have disturbed you."

He turned, wanting to leave as quickly as possible, but was halted by the general's harsh voice. "The woman. What did she look like?"

"Tall. Dark hair and brown eyes. About my age, I think. She is known as Mrs. Brown, though the doctor said that wasn't her real name." Dominic visualized that desperate face, trying to remember if there were any distinctive features. "She had a faint scar on her chin. Almost invisible." With a fingertip, he indicated on his own chin exactly how the scar ran.

Ames froze, expression stunned. "Dear God in heaven. She...Jena got that scar falling from a tree when she was six. It's her. *It's her!*"

149

His words hung in silence for an endless moment. Then he swung around and slammed a fist into the top railing, face contorted with anguish. "The bastard told me she was *dead*! That she'd died of smallpox while I was away, and had to be buried quickly. He...he showed me her grave in the family's private burial ground!"

Shocked, Dominic exclaimed, "Her husband faked her death?"

Collecting himself with visible effort, Ames spat out, "George Morton, may he rot in hell. How could any man betray his wife so horribly?"

"She told me that her husband had sent her to the asylum because she wasn't biddable. That she didn't agree with him." Dominic thought of his own father. "Some men cannot bear to be crossed. Perhaps Morton is one of them."

"But to say that she was mad! She was—is—as sane as I am. Though living as a prisoner with no hope of escape might drive her into madness." Ames's face darkened. "I warned her that Morton was a fortune hunter, but she wouldn't listen. He is evil. *Evil!*" The general gave a blood-chilling smile. "Before God, I swear that he will pay for this. But first I must bring Jena home." He pivoted and headed into the stables.

Concerned what the other man might do, Dominic followed. "Morton deserves a slow and painful death, but your daughter needs you alive, not swinging on a gibbet."

Ames began to saddle a tall gelding. "Oh, I don't intend to kill him. Much worse. I shall use the law to dismember him inch by inch. The estate he lives on was Jena's dowry. I shall take that, his good name, his so-called honor— everything he values. By the time I'm done, he'll wish I'd put a bullet into his wicked scheming brain."

Dominic might have felt sorry for Morton, if the man hadn't behaved so abominably. As the general led the gelding into the yard, he said, "Please send me a message at Warfield to let me know when your daughter is safely home."

"I shall." The general paused long enough to seize Dominic's hand in a crushing grip. "I've almost forgotten to thank you! I'm eternally in your debt, Maxwell." He pursed his lips. "Take Moonbeam for Lady Meriel. My gift."

Dominic gasped. "You can't do that with a horse so valuable!"

"You've just given me back my daughter. If you want the blood from my veins, you have but to ask," Ames said flatly. Then he swung onto the gelding and galloped off.

A little dazed, Dominic regarded the dainty gray mare. Ames had seemed quite sure of his mind, and pretty, well-behaved Moonbeam would be perfect for Meriel.

He turned to Pegasus, catching the horse's eye. "We're taking this little lady back to Warfield, and you will behave yourself on the journey. Do I make myself clear?"

Pegasus made a whuffling sound and swung his head away. "See that you remember that," Dominic said sternly.

As he opened the gate and went in to the mare, he wondered if Craythorne had known of Morton's scheme. No, the doctor's concern for patients and employees, his pride in his establishment, had been quite genuine. Impossible to imagine him cooperating voluntarily with a greedy, scheming husband.

Morton hadn't needed Craythorne's help; all he'd had to do was say sorrowfully that his wife was mad. Jena Morton looked like a strong-minded young woman, and her rage at the accusation became proof of her husband's charge. The bastard had been diabolically clever, for how does one prove sanity? Good behavior would be seen as merely the calm between storms. In fact, that was what Craythorne had told Dominic. Once she was committed, Jena had no chance of escape.

He stilled his tumbling thoughts before approaching the mare, for wild creatures, whether horses or mad girls, reacted to demeanor and tone of voice.

Extending one hand, he said softly, "Come with me, Moonbeam. You're going to a new home, and there's a moon maiden waiting."

Chapter 14

The elderly groom was delighted to welcome Moonbeam to the Warfield stables. As he brushed the mare to glossy perfection, he treated Dominic to fond reminiscences about the great days when Lord and Lady Grahame had been alive, and the stables had over-flowed with prime horseflesh. The groom also approved of the fact that Dominic pre-ferred to groom Pegasus himself, considering that the mark of a true horseman.

When he was finished, he returned to the house, and was immediately intercepted by Mrs. Rector, who asked, "What did you think of Bladenham?"

"A good institution of its kind, but no place for Meriel," he said flatly.

"I'm so glad that you agree with Lord Amworth." Mrs. Rector sighed. "Especially since she had a...a bad day."

Dominic frowned. "What does that mean?"

"This morning she attacked a fine old juniper hedge with her clippers. She's just hacking away furiously, with no rhyme or reason. It will take years for the damage to grow out." Mrs. Rector bit her lip. "She must have been upset by her uncle's visit, though I don't know if that was because he came, or because he left."

Or perhaps she was irritated by what had hap-pened with Dominic; she had not seemed happy when he put her out of his room the night before. "At least she didn't take the clippers to a person. Now, that would not be good."

The older woman smiled ruefully. "I shall remember to be grateful later. I always worry when she does something strange and destruc-tive, for fear her actions can be used as proof of dangerous madness."

Dominic thought of Jena Morton, who had been locked in an asylum on a man's word. Women were particularly vulnerable if the men who should protect them turned malicious, or venal, or even just wrongheaded. The only thing that had stood between Meriel and an asylum for all these years was Lord Amworth's determination. No wonder he wanted to see his niece in reliable hands as soon as possible.

"I'll go talk to Meriel. Not that I expect her to listen. Where is this hedge?"

"I'll take you." Mrs. Rector led him outside, then toward the east end of the gardens. He could hear the snap of pruning shears long before he saw his quarry.

He winced when he saw the embattled juniper hedge; Mrs. Rector had not exaggerated. Meriel had started at one end of the hedge and worked her way almost to the other end. A pity that Kamal had not been able to forestall her.

About two feet high, the hedge's purpose was to separate two sections of flower beds. Meriel knelt beside it, whacking at individual bushes. More than half the branches lay dying on the turf, exposing tangles of gnarled old trunks. The air was redolent with the tangy scent of fresh-cut evergreens.

Sensing the approach of visitors, she chopped off a branch, then looked up, fixing Dominic with a gimlet stare. He was startled by the light in her clear green eyes, which reminded him of a cat contemplating a tasty mouse.

Before he could confirm that fleeting impression, her gaze dropped to her work again. She studied the shrub in front of her, then raised the pruning shears and took off several thick twigs in rapid succession. Mrs. Rector gave a faint sigh.

Meriel wore her straw hat and long, thick gloves to protect her arms from scratches, so she wasn't totally lost to reason. Dominic approached her, saying, "I've brought you a present. Would you like to come see it?"

Not deigning to acknowledge him, she closed the jaws of her pruning shears around a branch, then frowned. After a moment, she withdrew the shears and took off a different branch. He asked, "What makes you choose one branch over another?"

She moved to her right and lopped off a piece on the adjacent juniper. Wryly he thought that he might as well ask Meriel's cat why it slept under a particular nearby bush, and not the one next to it. He'd get as much answer.

His gaze moved over the butchered hedge, and suddenly something clicked in his mind. Slowly he began walking along the line of heavily pruned shrubs, looking not at what was gone, but what was left. Contorted knots of trunk anchored deep in the earth. Craggy branches that hugged the ground for yards before twisting sharply toward the sun.

"Mrs. Rector, Meriel isn't cutting at random," he said, intrigued. "She started with a hedge so bland and ordinary it was almost invisible, and transformed it like a surgeon whose scalpel cuts away the flesh to reveal the underlying skeleton. In this case, she's chopping away the clutter of twigs and small branches to reveal the basic structure of the junipers. Look at how bold and powerful the shapes are now that we can see them."

He sketched one hand above a pair of gnarled branches that crisscrossed in a brutal struggle for space and light. Another branch dived under them, then doubled dramatically back on itself before opening into greenery. The shrubs were like miniature versions of the wind-tortured trees found on a stormy shore.

Even more, the junipers reminded him of pictures in a book that belonged to his brother. Kyle enjoyed all things Oriental, and had somehow acquired a volume of Chinese prints. The stark elemental strength of the trees depicted in the pictures found robust life in Meriel's hedge. "The bushes look a bit raw now, but by autumn there will be enough new growth to balance the trunks and the greenery properly."

Mrs. Rector's brows drew together. "I...I think I see what you mean. The effect is really quite interesting." She bit her lip. "Beautiful but mad."

More potential evidence of Meriel's lunacy, in other words. "Is it mad to see the world in a fresh way? Artists do. Of course, sometimes they are considered mad, too. But without that kind of madness, the world would be a poorer place. Meriel is an artist of the garden. She has created a fresh kind of beauty, for those who choose to see."

He caught a movement from the corner of his eye, and glanced over to find Meriel looking up at him, her pruning shears still. Their gazes met, and a jolt shot through him. As clearly as if she spoke the words aloud, he sensed her saying, *"You understand."*

The impact was more powerful than if they'd physically touched. He felt, for an instant, as if he'd entered her world, a magical place unlike his own mundane existence.

Then she dropped her eyes, and the moment was gone. He was left with a yearning to connect with her again. To share her vision, be transformed by her magic.

And that would be a disastrous mistake. The closer he drew to Meriel, the greater the likelihood of trouble when the real Lord Maxwell arrived to claim his bride. Dominic had no business looking into her eyes and seeing wonders.

He turned abruptly and offered Mrs. Rector his arm. "Let me escort you back to the house." And on the way, he could regain his self-control. Then he would introduce Meriel to Moonbeam, and give her something new to engage her attention.

He had a swift mental picture of Meriel galloping the mare across the park. He hastily buried the image when he realized she was riding like Lady Godiva, clad only in her flowing silver hair.

That way madness lay.

Hands shaking, Meriel began to prune the last juniper. He understood. *He understood!* Most people went through life half-blind, seeing only what they expected, but *he recognized the power and beauty around him.*

She stole a quick glance as he walked away with Mrs. Rector, admiring the smooth swing of his steps, the power in his broad shoulders. Male strength, at ease in his own body in a way more animal than human. Points of crimson light sparkled deep in the energy that surrounded him. Red for desire. He wanted her, she was sure of it. But how was she to lure him into mating?

Distracted, she chopped off a branch that should have stayed, and cursed herself for her carelessness. Yearning and pruning didn't mix. More carefully, she removed a series of branchlets that obscured the stark grandeur of the juniper.

A strange thought struck her. He lived in the world very easily, it seemed, yet he had also come fully alive in hers. If he could live in two worlds, might she also?

The idea sparked a flare of nightmare images. Annihilating flames, screaming horses and humans, the Dark One whose torch had set the world ablaze. Terror exploded in her mind, shaking her like a weasel snapping the neck of a mouse. She dropped her shears and folded over, gasping, arms wrapped around her middle against the pain.

Ginger came awake and appeared at her

side, pressing his broad feline head into her ribs as he gave a low miaow. Gratefully she picked him up and held his warm body close as he rumbled into purrs. Cats could live in two worlds. Perhaps Renbourne could also. But not her. Not now. Not ever.

After returning Mrs. Rector to the house and checking that all was ready in the stables, Dominic went to collect Meriel. She had just finished pruning the last juniper, and was rather stiffly rising to her feet.

"Are you ready for your present?" Dominic asked. As usual, he had no idea to what extent Meriel registered his presence. She gave a catlike stretch to loosen up. Trying not to stare at the flex of her lithe body, he touched her elbow gently. "Come."

To his relief, she fell into step beside him. He hadn't been quite sure what to do if she paid him no heed. Picking her up and carrying her would hardly be suitable, and besides, she'd probably scratch his eyes out.

He surreptitiously watched her as they walked. She looked a little tired from her day's work, and long strands of flaxen hair had escaped from the braid to drift around her face, but she appeared quite composed. Sane. Chopping up that hedge hadn't been a mad start; she'd probably been planning it for weeks.

The stables were fragrant with hay, the dim light a pleasant respite from the afternoon sun. Dominic had told the groom to put

Moonbeam into a large box stall at the far end of the building, so he guided Meriel along the central aisle. "Down here."

Seeing visitors, Moonbeam moved to the door of the stall and stretched out her neck, whickering sociably. The groom had combed out the long white mane and tail until they were as glossy as Meriel's hair, then playfully tied a blue ribbon into her forelock. A horse fit for a fairy-tale princess. Dominic explained, "Properly speaking, this gift is not from me, but from a neighbor of yours, General Ames."

He watched with pleasure as Meriel's eyes widened. Then, to his shock, she made a wordless cry and spun around. Her voice carried the blind fear of the time he had tried to take her outside of Warfield.

As she bolted toward the door, he reacted from pure instinct, stepping into her path to block her escape. She slammed into him so hard that he lost his balance and fell backward into a pile of straw intended for bedding, Meriel clutched against him.

Sprigs of straw flew around them as she struggled to free herself. He wrapped his arms tight, immobilizing her. "Don't run, Meriel! Not this time. Running doesn't help."

She was like a trapped songbird, fragile and frantic of heartbeat. Why the devil was she so upset? Though she had been nervous of Pegasus when he took her riding, there had been nothing like this wild panic. Softly he repeated, "Don't run, sweeting. You're safe here with me."

160

Her struggles stilled, but she shivered uncontrollably, as if racked with fever. Settling into the straw, he pulled her across his lap and pressed her head into his shoulder as he held her close. Silky hair spilled over his fingers, gossamer as butterfly wings.

Where to begin? Remembering what Ames said, he asked, "Are you upset because Moonbeam looks like the pony you had in India?"

A shudder ran through her. Guessing that he was on the right track, he continued in his most soothing voice, "That silver gray is a rare color in England; you probably haven't seen a horse like that since you left India." Particularly since she hadn't left Warfield for more than fifteen years. "Does Moonbeam remind you of losing your parents?"

There were no tears in her stark green eyes, but she made a choked noise and hid her face against him. He tried to imagine what that catastrophic night had been like for a small child. The minor rajah's palace, scented with the flowers and spices of the East. Then a sudden fierce night attack. "Battle is terrifying even for experienced soldiers. Ear-numbing guns, screams of fear and pain, perhaps fire. Your mother and father killed, along with all the servants. Then you were abducted by savage strangers, and alone."

As he tried to visualize what had happened, he had an eerie sense of connection with her past. Probably she'd been carried off on horseback by a stinking barbarian, crying desperately for the mother she would never see

161

again. Christ, what a horror for a sheltered child!

He'd been appropriately dismayed when he first heard Meriel's story, but the events had been long ago and far away, and they'd happened to someone he had not yet met. Now that he knew her, he *felt* her experience in his very marrow. "Poor sweeting," he whispered. "So much horror, then being held captive in an alien land. Is that why you stopped talking—because there was no one who understood your words?"

Even if she was treated kindly in her captivity, she had been isolated, deprived of the comfort of her own people, locked in her head with memories of destruction. No wonder she had retreated to a private world and never come out again. Withdrawal had been necessary for her survival. He was as sure of that as he was of his own name.

And she had been alone ever since, trapped inside a fragile bubble of safety adrift in a sea of terrors. With bone-deep intensity, he wanted to free her from the scars of her past. Though once withdrawal had protected her, now that private world had become a prison. He wanted her to be free, not for Kyle's sake but for her own.

How could he reach her?

An infected physical wound was lanced to let decaying matter escape. He needed to touch her fears, then somehow lance them so they would flow away and no longer torment her. Perhaps he could achieve that by speaking of his own terrors. To speak of his wartime experiences was to reveal that he was Dominic, not Kyle, but it was unlikely she would ever realize that. Besides, the small risk involved was worth it. Though she might not understand his words, she might recognize the pain in his voice and know that she was not alone.

"Once I was a soldier, Meriel." His father had decreed that as a younger son Dominic must go into either the church or the army. Since he didn't fancy himself a vicar, he chose the military. Kyle had been furious and tried to bully his brother into studying with him at Cambridge. But that was not the particular pain Dominic meant to share today. "You must have seen lots of soldiers in India. Your uncle was one."

She twisted nervously at his words. "Shhh..." he murmured. "I'll keep you safe, Meriel, I swear it."

When she was calm again, he continued, "I chose the cavalry because I was horse-mad. I was just a boy at the time, only seventeen. I thought war was a great adventure. I would become a dashing hero, and be much admired by the ladies. Lord, I was a fool, and doubly a fool for being delighted when Napoleon returned from exile, and did his damnedest to set Europe ablaze once more."

He had the sense that Meriel was listening. Did she really understand the words? At least she was responding, even if only to his voice.

"Which is how I ended up as a grass-green cornet—that's the lowest rank of cavalry officer—on the plains of Waterloo. The greatest battle in history, perhaps. My first and last taste of combat." Words caught in his throat. He'd told no one what that day had been like. Once he could have told Kyle, but by then they were already too estranged for him to admit weakness even to his brother. Especially to his brother.

"I thought I'd be nervous when facing battle, but I didn't expect the gut-wrenching terror that would turn my bowels to water." He swallowed, hard. "I was frightened of everything. Death, of course, but even more of slow agonizing death, of having my belly ripped out by a bullet and dying in the mud for days. Of seeing friends die before my eyes, and being unable to help. Of surviving so horribly mangled that my life was ruined forever, and I would be a helpless cripple."

In his worst nightmares, he'd imagined himself blind and paralyzed at Dornleigh, kept alive from pity and family obligation, too helpless even to kill himself. Suppressing a shudder, he continued, "Most of all I feared that I would prove to be a coward, so despised that men would spit when they heard my name. That I would break and run, and cost the lives of other, better men."

His breath came in hard, shallow gasps as the events of that fatal day sprang to horrifying life. "Waterloo was hell come to earth, Meriel. The stink of powder and the screams of dying men. The pounding of the guns and eyes blinded by smoke. Not knowing what was going on. *Not knowing*. In some ways, that was worst of all."

He stroked her back with a damp palm. "I didn't disgrace myself, thank God, though I certainly was no hero. A wise and canny sergeant named Finn saved me from causing damage with my inexperience. I was able to master my fear enough to charge when the commands came down."

He fell silent, remembering. "I'll never forget the excitement of galloping toward the French, the thunder of hooves, guns shaking the ground like an earthquake. There was a mad rapture to the charge, and in some ways that was most frightening of all, because that crazy pleasure is why men continue to go to war." Cutting short the digression, he said tersely, "I don't know how many times we charged. A lot. But I survived, and began to think I might make it through the battle after all. Then...then..."

He stopped, unable to continue. Meriel's small, strong hand crept out and came to rest on top of his with unexpected tenderness. Somehow her shaking had been transferred to him. "My horse, Ajax, was struck. He was a wonderful fellow, strong and steady as Sergeant Finn. I'd already promised Ajax a lifetime of green meadows and oats for carrying me so well. And then on the last charge of the day, he was hit by French bullets and went down. And I went down underneath him."

The mud had saved him, reducing the impact of being crushed beneath a half-ton horse. He stared sightlessly at the window, not seeing the fertile gardens outside. "I was knocked witless for a time. When I woke, there was nothing around me but dead men and slaughtered horses. One...one of the men was Sergeant Finn."

He drew a shaky breath. It had seemed so bloody damned unfair that he had survived when a brave man like Finn had died. He'd sent money to Finn's family later, though it was poor compensation for what Finn had done for him.

Wanting to get this over, he said tightly, "I could hear moans and screams of anguish, but the cannon smoke lay on the field so heavily that I might have been alone in purgatory. Except that Ajax was alive, barely. Dying in agony, his blood saturating me. I could feel his pain, yet he never made a sound except ghastly bubbling noises as he tried to breathe. I could do nothing, not even find a knife to...to slit his throat."

Meriel turned her face until the soft, smooth skin of her forehead rested against his cheek. He felt a pulse between them and didn't know if it was hers or his. "I was trapped there for two days. Both nights looters came by. The first night they tore the silver lace from my coat; the next night they took the coat, but they made no attempt to free me, though I begged them for help."

That had been the ultimate degradation— to lose whatever claim he had to dignity in frantic, futile pleas. "I was almost dead of thirst by the time our men found me. Ajax had died by then, of course." The warm, intelligent beast who had carried him so well transformed into cold, dead flesh.

There had been flies.

"I had cuts and scrapes and cracked ribs, but the real damage was to my mind. I thought I'd never ride again. Bloody hell, I didn't want to ever see another horse, even though I'd loved them all my life."

Meriel's fingers slid into his hair, caressing. She was offering the comfort she had never received herself. He closed his eyes against a swift sting of tears. Though he had deliberately chosen to offer his pain to her, he...hadn't expected it to hurt quite so much.

He took a dozen deep, slow breaths. "What eventually pulled me out was the company of the friends in my regiment. Not that we talked about the horrors of Waterloo, but just knowing that others had been there, had shared the same excitement and fear, helped me get my feet under me again. Though the memories didn't vanish, they retreated to a place where they didn't bother me anymore." Except now, when he had deliberately opened the door to where fear lived.

"If you could talk, sweeting, you could tell of your private horrors. Perhaps that would make them go away," he said quietly, his breath stirring her silky hair. "But even if you can't speak, know that you are not alone now."

For the space of a dozen heartbeats, she didn't move. Then she pulled away from his relaxed embrace and turned to face him, kneeling in the straw. Her gaze met his, sober and direct. Or perhaps determined was a better description. Because she was petite and ethereally slight, it was easy to think of her as a fragile, spun sugar angel. But what he saw in her expression now was pure steel.

She reached out and cupped his face with cool, slim fingers. Giving strength, or receiving it? Then she rose smoothly, brushed her hands down her skirt in an unconscious admission of nerves, and slowly walked to Moonbeam.

Dominic's heart jumped into his throat when he saw Meriel approach the mare. Praying that Moonbeam would be her usual sweet self, he got to his feet slowly so as not to distract either girl or horse.

Meriel came to a dead halt, her body rigid. Voice conversational, he said, "Horses like to know who's in charge. Even the best of them challenge new people, so you need to establish yourself as Moonbeam's mistress from the start. Approach with confidence. Head up, shoulders back. If she crowds you, don't back off."

Meriel lifted her chin. After drawing a deep breath, she moved within touching distance of the mare. Moonbeam promptly stretched her neck and butted the girl's ribs. The gesture was friendly, but also a test. Luckily, though Meriel flinched, she didn't retreat. With stiff fingers, she skimmed her palm down Moonbeam's neck once, then again. Gradually the tension faded from her body.

Dominic released the breath he'd been holding. "She likes you. Here, give her this." He took a lump of sugar from his pocket. "Flat on your palm."

Horses had large teeth and strong jaws, and Dominic wouldn't have blamed Meriel if she refused, but warily she offered the sugar. The mare delicately lapped it up. Meriel's face lit with an enchanting smile. Apparently the link between silvery gray horse and her parents' death had been broken. Now she could appreciate Moonbeam for the beautiful beast she was rather than seeing her as a symbol of disaster.

Wanting to build on this success, he said, "According to General Ames you were an excellent rider when you were a child, and I think that's something one never forgets. Shall we saddle up and go for a quiet ride?" There would never be a better time; he'd ridden from Holliwell Grange on Moonbeam to check her moods and paces, so the mare had all the fidgets worked out of her.

Meriel frowned. After a long moment, she turned on her heel and walked away. Dominic suppressed a pang of disappointment; he'd been hoping for too much, too soon.

Then he realized that Meriel was heading for the tack room.

Chapter 15

How could she have forgotten the freedom found only on horseback? But that had been buried with so much else from the Time Before. She signaled Moonbeam into a gallop, laughing with pure delight as they raced through the park. She could almost believe she rode beloved Daisy, dead these eighteen years, but Daisy had never been so sleek and swift.

Deliberately she let grief wash through her, calling up memories of the terrified whinnying that ripped through the night when the stables exploded into flame. She'd recognized Daisy's scream, higher-pitched than those of the full-size horses.

Then, after a silent good-bye, she released her sadness to dissolve in the Warfield winds.

Gradually she slowed the mare's headlong pace to allow him to catch up with her. She owed Renbourne much, not only for this soaring joy but for his halting, anguished revelations. She'd believed herself uniquely cursed, a weakling, for all of those around her had mastered their lives. Not like her, tossed like thistledown in a tempest.

He cantered easily toward her, his expression relaxed and warm. She would not have recognized the sorrow in him if he had not revealed it voluntarily. It made her wonder how often grief was concealed by others. If a man like him could ache so deeply, hidden sorrows must be common indeed.

If she had needed more proof that he was meant for her, she had it now.

Dominic watched Meriel race down the hill, her wind-whipped braid flaring behind her. Hard to believe that she hadn't ridden a horse since she was a child. Ames hadn't exaggerated when he talked about her tearing across the plains like an Afghan bandit. She was a natural on horseback.

Dominic urged Pegasus down the hill in her wake. She'd chosen a man's saddle from the tack room, and totally ignored his suggestion that she find a pair of boots, or at least shoes. The lack didn't appear to bother her in the least.

Radiating delight, she reined Moonbeam in and turned the mare to face Dominic as he approached. With her bare feet and skirt hiked to her knees, she looked a proper hoyden. But what mattered was that she looked—unafraid.

He felt a rush of pleasure at the sight. For too long she had been allowed to drift because no one expected anything of her. What might she become with the right encouragement?

Recklessly deciding to try one last hurdle, he said, "I need to ride to the home farm and talk to the steward about possible work for Jem Brown, the poacher. Will you come with me?"

The delicate color drained from her face, leaving it bone white. She started to turn Moonbeam away. He caught the mare's bridle. "We would be leaving the park, but if we use the east gate, on the other side of that hill, we'll never be off Warfield land. It will be a very short visit, and the only people you might see will be your employees."

Moonbeam stirred restlessly as Meriel's hands slackened in uncertainty. But at least she wasn't running away.

Hopeful, he released the mare's bridle. "I won't force you. But if you come, I swear that you'll be safe."

He set Pegasus into a walk toward the east gate without looking back. There was no sound of a following horse. He released his breath, not really surprised. She'd had a demanding day already. Asking her to leave Warfield was simply too much.

Then he heard a faint jingle of harness behind him, and the rhythm of trotting hooves. He wanted to whoop aloud with pleasure. He refrained so as not to startle the horses, but he gave a welcoming smile when she brought her mount even with his.

They reached the east gate. A pair of doors set into a stone archway, it was secured with a heavy bar. Dominic dismounted to lift the bar and swing the doors open. Then he waited for Meriel to ride through.

She balked. As she sat unmoving on Moonbeam's back, he sensed the coiled tension behind her expressionless face. What seemed so simple to him—riding outside the park— was for her a barrier of shattering height. Worse than being ordered to charge a French regiment, because at least a soldier was surrounded by his fellows. Meriel looked very alone. Had been alone for most of her life. Dominic could be with her physically, but she must overcome her demons herself.

Unable to bear her inward struggle any longer, he was about to tell her he would go alone when she urged her mount forward in a slow walk. Sensing her rider's anxiety, the mare went through the gate as warily as if she were walking on a rickety wooden bridge. But they made it. Together, they made it.

"Well done, Meriel!" Awed by her courage, he closed the door without latching it so they could return the same way. Then he remounted for the ride to the home farm. Dominic hadn't visited before, but he knew the location from the Warfield maps. He viewed the fertile fields with pleasure as they followed a grassy lane that led to the farmstead. The steward, one John Kerr according to Mrs. Rector, knew his job.

The farmstead was laid out rather like Holliwell Grange. As they entered a yard enclosed by a rambling house and outbuildings, Dominic spotted a boy of about ten sitting on a bench outside the stables, industriously cleaning a saddle.

"Good afternoon," Dominic said amiably. "Is Mr. Kerr available?"

The boy's gaze went over Pegasus with approval. "He's in the estate office, sir. I'll get him for you."

Then the boy saw Meriel, and his eyes widened. She was studying the farmyard with interest, but when she became aware of the child's gaze her face shuttered.

Hardly able to tear his gaze from her, the boy went into the estate office. Dominic glanced around the yard and saw that a woman, probably Mrs. Kerr, was looking out an upper window of the house. A young girl dressed as a maid appeared at a ground floor window, and was quickly joined by another.

Dominic muttered a mental oath. He should have anticipated this. Lady Meriel Grahame, the mad heiress of Warfield, must be more myth than reality in the neighborhood. Of course her dependents would be fascinated.

He tried to see her as if for the first time rather than as the girl he'd come to know. With her wild hair, eccentric costume and bare feet, and her refusal to meet anyone's eyes, he feared that she fulfilled her reputation for lunacy. He wanted to shout that she wasn't like that, that she was bright and perceptive and had the soul of an artist, but doing so would merely make him appear equally mad.

By the time the steward emerged from the office, almost a dozen people were watching from various vantages around the farmstead. In the middle of the yard, Meriel held Moonbeam so still, they looked like a statue. Dominic kept a watchful eye on her, praying that she wouldn't bolt under all the attention.

Mr. Kerr, a solid man with shrewd eyes, said, "Would you be Lord Maxwell?"

"I am. A pleasure to meet you, Mr. Kerr." Dominic offered his hand.

The steward gave him a firm handshake as he studied Dominic with the interest of a man summing up a possible future employer. No doubt everyone in the neighborhood knew of "Maxwell's" visit to Warfield. Kerr had probably been waiting for a call.

Dominic continued, "Have you ever met Lady Meriel?"

Kerr allowed his gaze to go to Meriel with unabashed interest. "We met once when Lord Amworth took me to Warfield, but I doubt she'd remember. Welcome to Swallow Farm, my lady."

Probably when they'd met the first time she had ignored the steward as she ignored most people. She was staring across the yard now, as if willing her surroundings to vanish. But—she wasn't running.

"Yesterday I met a young man called Jem Brown who is in dire need of work," Dominic explained. "I took the liberty of suggesting that he call on you tomorrow. I don't know if you can use another laborer, but he looked willing. If you don't need him, perhaps you know someone in the area who does."

"The haying will begin soon, so I can use more hands," Kerr replied. "If the lad is a hard worker, there's a place for him here."

"Thank you, Mr. Kerr. That's very kind of you." Dominic saw the sardonic glint in the steward's eye at the comment. Both of them knew perfectly well that the steward would hire anyone recommended by Lady Meriel's potential husband. Now it was up to Jem to behave himself and give up poaching. Or at least have the sense not to get caught.

"Would you like a tour of the home farm? Or the tenant farms?" Kerr offered. "The tenants would be delighted to meet you."

"Not today, thank you." Dominic glanced at Meriel. The sooner he got her away from here, the better. Besides, as much as he would enjoy a tour, it wouldn't do to let a sharp-eyed fellow like Kerr get close enough to know him well. "Perhaps another time."

After an exchange of farewells, Dominic turned his horse to leave. Instantly Meriel and Moonbeam fell into step beside him. She maintained her taut control as they walked from the farmyard. A dozen people waited outside, hungry for a glimpse of the mythical Lady Meriel. How the devil had they gotten word of her presence so quickly?

Head high and back ramrod straight, she rode past the onlookers like a queen. Dominic gave a sigh of relief. She had done it.

His relief was premature. As soon as they were clear of the farmstead and watchers, Moonbeam took off like an angry hornet. He set Pegasus in pursuit, regretting that he had coaxed Meriel into this expedition.

A barred gate crossed the lane ahead. Earlier Dominic had opened it so they could ride through. This time—dear God, she wasn't slowing down, she was going to jump it! A tall gate, on a strange horse, and a rider who hadn't been on horseback since she was a child. Had she done any jumping when she was so young?

He pounded after them, heart in his mouth. If Moonbeam hit the top bar, both horse and rider might break their necks.

The mare thundered headlong toward the gate. She was in a good position, she was lifting into the air...

Horse and rider soared over the gate, making a perfect landing on the other side. Torn between relief and a desire to wring Meriel's neck, Dominic took Pegasus over the gate as well, but he didn't catch up with her until she reached the gate to the park. There she reined in her mount and waited for him, demure as a pair of kid gloves.

"You ride like a centaur," he said tartly. "And almost stopped my heart in the process."

Her eyes widened with such innocence that he knew she was baiting him. Grinning, he dismounted and opened the gate. "After what you've achieved today, I suppose you're entitled to your fun. But if I have gray hairs tomorrow, it will be your fault."

She took off for home at an easy trot, her enchanting laughter floating behind her. At times like this, he was almost sure that she understood him.

When they reached the stables, Dominic dismounted from Pegasus and led him inside. Regally Meriel rode Moonbeam into the building with plenty of room to spare between her head and the ceiling.

"Just a moment and I'll help you dismount," he said to Meriel as he removed Pegasus's saddle.

Her brows arched with delicate scorn. He chuckled, feeling as if they were having a real conversation. "I know you can get down easily enough, sprite, but it's time you learned how a lady behaves. You'll enjoy being a hoyden more if you know how outrageous your conduct is."

Though the last leg of their ride had been slow enough to cool the horses, they still needed to be rubbed down. He'd give Meriel a quick lesson. While she had servants for menial work, a true horsewoman must understand how to care for a horse herself.

He led Pegasus into the stall and temporarily threw a blanket over him. Then he went to Moonbeam and raised his arms to assist Meriel down. "I don't suppose you were taught grooming when you were five years old, so we'll have a lesson before dinner."

She swung her leg over the mare, then rested her hands on his shoulders and dismounted. But she didn't settle lightly on the ground like a seasoned gentlewoman rider. Instead, she came into his arms like a woman running to her lover. He turned rigid, instinctively catching her against him. This was *not* what he had intended—but dear God, she felt so good!

Torn between wanting to hold her and knowing he must let her go, he reluctantly loosened his grip. A proper lady would have stepped away. Meriel slowly, deliberately, slid down the front of his body, every supple curve impressing itself on him like flame.

Then she turned her face up to his, her

eyes clear and intent. He wanted to kiss those soft, parted lips. He wanted to loosen her hair so he could bury his face in its shimmering magnificence. Most of all, he wanted to make love to her until they were both senseless with fulfillment.

As he stood frozen, she touched his lips with her fingertips in unmistakable invitation, a faint smile on her face. Helplessly he drew her index finger into his mouth, caressing it with his tongue. She began sliding her finger in and out with natural sensuality. How could something so simple be so arousing?

Because everything about her aroused him. God help him, it was impossible to deny any longer how much he desired her. This wild woman sprite affected him, body and soul, as no one ever had before.

Shakily reminding himself of all the reasons that he mustn't continue this, he caught her hand and moved it away. "Meriel..."

Before he could say more, she slipped her arms around his neck and leaned into him. He retreated, and she followed with the sweet insistence of a puppy swarming up her owner, seeking treats.

He halted when his back flattened against the wall, but she kept going, walking up onto his boots. Her small bare feet scarcely dented the leather, but she gained several inches of height.

Then she kissed him full on the mouth, her hands stroking his neck and into his hair. Her lips were unskilled, but marvelously soft. Questing.

Common sense vanished, and he kissed her back. She tasted like wild strawberries, as fresh and luscious as the springtime. Small delicate bones, but strong, so strong. He stroked her back, cupping her hips, drawing her against him.

"You are so lovely," he murmured into her mouth. Then he kissed her throat. Her head fell back, and she gave a breathy sigh. She was an innocent with an appetite as ancient as Lilith, the first temptress. He was aching hard, almost mindless with desire as his body throbbed against hers.

He was reaching for her breast when a solid head butted into his ribs, jarring him from his sensual haze. He blinked dizzily and saw that Moonbeam, abandoned by her rider, was trying to eat his coat. Specifically, his pocket. He gave an unsteady laugh. "You want some more sugar, don't you, girl?"

Not daring to look into Meriel's eyes, he firmly moved her to one side so that her toes wouldn't get mashed by steel-shod hooves. Then he dug a lump of sugar from his coat pocket with shaking fingers and offered it to the mare. She happily slurped it from his palm, then gave him a melting gaze in hopes of more.

Trying to pretend that scorching embrace had never happened, he caught Moonbeam's reins. "You and Pegasus need to be rubbed down."

He led the mare to her stall, thinking that he owed her a whole loaf of sugar for saving him from temporary insanity. Christ, what could be madder than wanting to lie with his brother's future wife? The potential for damage to everyone involved was horrifying. Despite Meriel's innocent enthusiasm, she couldn't possibly understand the implications of what she was inviting him to do. The physical aspects of sex were relatively simple. It was the emotional and moral consequences that raised hell.

Damnation, why wasn't Kyle here, wooing his bride himself?

His best efforts at control could not quell the throbbing in his groin, or the desire to teach Meriel what she was so eager to learn. He glanced over his shoulder. She stood where he had left her, fists clenched at her sides and her eyes dark with passion. He might be constrained by multiple reasons to keep his distance, but she wasn't.

She wanted him. And gods above, if he had a grain of sense he would leave Warfield immediately, for he wasn't sure he would have the strength to refuse her again.

Chapter 16

Kyle knocked lightly, then entered Constancia's cabin. She lay on the small chaise, gazing into a hand mirror as she applied a faint blush of rouge to her cheeks with a hare's foot. When Kyle entered, she made a rueful face. "Alas, querido, you have caught me. Isn't it amazing how vanity persists even at the end of life? One of the seven deadly sins, and enough to condemn me to the fire even if I hadn't committed most of the other sins as well."

Glad she was strong enough to be concerned with her appearance, he kissed one thin, perfume-scented hand before taking the chair opposite the chaise. "Why shouldn't you have a care for your looks, La Paloma? After all, your face has been your fortune."

She sighed, her animation fading to reveal underlying fatigue. "And a mixed fortune it has been. My curse, and my survival."

"Your beauty a curse?" The thought saddened him, for he had taken such pleasure in her classical loveliness.

She stroked the chased silver back of the mirror, expression brooding. "I had a sister, only a year older than I. As little girls we were very close, but as we grew, we became... competitive. She was pretty, but not so pretty as me. And I, shameless creature, flaunted my beauty. My family was of the *hidalgo* class, rather like your gentry, but I had larger plans. I boasted of the grand husband I would have, the wealth and jewels that would be mine, because surely my father would marry me into the nobility. My mother encouraged my dreams, for my success would be her triumph."

He was surprised but intrigued, since Constancia never referred to her past. The bare outlines that he knew were common knowledge. Hoping to encourage the flow of reminiscence, he observed, "It's natural for mothers to take pride in their daughters."

"But it should not be done at the price of another daughter." She rested her head against the arm of the chaise, her expression distant. "My sister, María Magdalena, was better and sweeter than I. She lacked my ambitions and wished for us to be friends, but I made that difficult. Then war came, and my family was destroyed. I heard my sister screaming as the...the soldiers assaulted her." Constancia's eyes closed and pain spasmed across her face. "Her screams stopped when they cut her throat."

He stared, shocked to his marrow at her flat recitation. "You heard her die?"

"Oh, yes." She smiled bitterly. "I also was ravished that day, but because of my beauty, an officer claimed me for himself. He thought me too lovely to kill. So instead, after he and his brother officers dishonored me, I was left to starve by the ruins of my home and the bodies of my family."

He took her hand, wishing helplessly that he could change the past. "Querida, I am so sorry. No one should have to endure such wickedness. The wonder is that you didn't go mad."

Her eyes opened, dark and piercing as she looked directly at him. "When the hand of God strikes, there is little that a mere mortal can do. But I have never forgiven myself for the fact that my sister and I died estranged, and the fault was mine. I would give every valuable I ever possessed for the chance to tell her how much I loved her."

He understood then why she was revealing so much of herself. Withdrawing his hand from hers, he said dryly, "You're giving me advice about my brother, aren't you?"

"There is no time for subtlety. One day María Magdalena and I were sharing a maid and I was taunting her with the fine marriage offer my father had received. The next day she and the world I knew were dead." Constancia swallowed, her throat painfully thin. "I have sometimes thought she died so quickly as the reward for her good soul. I, being wicked, was not granted that grace."

Her words created pain deep inside him. "Has your life been so dreadful that you wish you had died then?"

Her eyes softened. "There have been compensations, mi corazón. I have had better fortune than I deserved. But it is not the life I would have chosen."

He was a fool for taking her words personally; of course she wouldn't have chosen the tragedy she had endured. But without it, they would never have met. Selfishly, he wanted her to be glad to have known him in spite of all that implied.

She interrupted his thoughts to ask, "If you returned to England and found your brother suddenly dead, would you be satisfied with the state of your relations with him?"

No. The answer was instant. He'd always thought the tension between him and Dom was merely a phase. Eventually his brother would start acting sensibly, and they would be friends again. Yet—life was uncertain. If something happened to Dominic, would he feel the kind of guilt Constancia felt about María Magdalena?

Not liking the answer, he said defensively, "You said that your sister wished to be friends. My brother has shown no wish to rebuild our relationship. He persists in the same kind of bullheaded idiocy that he has shown since we were boys."

"It is rare for only one person to be at fault, mi corazón," Constancia murmured. "Can you truly say that all the trouble between you is caused by him?"

Angrily he got to his feet and walked to a port. Outside, a squall spattered rain into a pewter gray sea. "I've always done my part, but Dominic persists in wasting his life. He could have joined me at Cambridge and studied for the church, but he wouldn't."

He had hoped so much that his brother would agree. They would have become close again. Dom's refusal had been like a slap in the face. "My father bought him a commission in the cavalry. He became bored and sold out after a year. He could travel to the ends of the earth, learning and exploring and writing me letters of what he has seen. Instead, he spends his days on the shallowest of pleasures. If I had his opportunities..." He cut off

185

the bitter words, hating the resentment he heard in his voice.

"Most men would say that the opportunities are all yours," she said shrewdly. "Do you envy his freedom? Despise him for not using it the same way you would?"

He flinched as if she had struck him. Of course he didn't envy Dominic! The power, the wealth, came to the elder son. Kyle had been born for that. Why should he be jealous of the fact that his brother was...free?

He closed his eyes, feeling as if he were choking. Why should he want to weep when he was the lucky one?

Chapter 17

By the time Dominic had finished rubbing down the horses, belatedly aided by the elderly groom, he barely had time to wash and change before dinner. He was rather glad that Meriel skipped the meal; he would have had trouble eating with her sitting across from him, looking alarmingly desirable.

Her presence was felt in the centerpieces, however. The splendid globes of rhododendrons might have been picked by anyone, but only Meriel would think to arrange the blooms in masses that spilled from a battered tin watering can in a lavender river.

As he took his seat, chatting easily with Mrs. Marks, he studied the flower arrangement.

"The centerpiece is like Meriel's juniper hedge—unconventional, but quite lovely in its own way. Look at the contrast of the flamboyant, colorful rhododendrons and the well-used, workaday watering can. Really quite dramatic and interesting, don't you think?"

He flushed a little when he saw Mrs. Marks's startled expression. She must be wondering if Meriel's madness was contagious. Mrs. Rector, though, tilted her head to one side reflectively. "I believe I see what you mean, my lord. The combination is quite intriguing. Though I must admit that I would prefer a pretty china vase."

"The arrangement is certainly original," Mrs. Marks conceded. "But perhaps better suited to the kitchen than the center of a mahogany table."

Dominic didn't argue the point. Before coming to Warfield, he would have agreed wholeheartedly. Unthinkingly. Meriel was changing the way he viewed the world. He took a sip of wine. "Did you know that Meriel can ride?"

The subject, along with the other events of the day, kept the conversation lively until the three of them were ready to retire to their beds.

After Renbourne's rejection, Meriel fled the stables, furious and humiliated. He'd been willing at first. What was wrong with her that he would not mate? Damn the man!

But the fault surely lay with her. She'd

watched the birds and field creatures, and seen that female readiness triggered the male response. She must not be fully in season yet. Though if she were any more ready, she'd burst into flame!

Seeing Roxana dozing in the shade of an arbor, Meriel dropped onto the wooden seat and inhaled the scent of the roses that twined around and above her. The dog sleepily rested her head on Meriel's foot, the shaggy fur tickling her toes.

As she scratched the dog's ears, she told herself that when she had more experience in mating, she would know what to expect. She would know the right movements, the signals, to bring him to her. Useful though it was to watch falcons and foxes, they could not show her the rituals humans required.

She frowned, thinking of one human custom that she might try. And if that didn't work—well, there were methods she'd observed in the zenana. They required much effort, but surely no man living could resist them.

The mehndi patterns had darkened from light orange to rust red. Dominic studied the design in the mirror, glad he had dismissed Morrison before removing his shirt. He had no wish to see speculation in the valet's eyes.

Yawning, he prepared to dowse the lamp and climb into bed. He pulled back the coverlet, then stopped. Nestled between the two pillows was a ribbon-tied nosegay.

He picked up the spray of blossoms, knowing

it had to be from Meriel. Two small carnations, one white, one red. There was also one of the lavender-tinted wild pansies called heartsease, and a narrow willow leaf. A pretty little arrangement, as unusual as everything else Meriel created.

He inhaled the fragrance, which was dominated by the spicy carnation scents. There was something wickedly erotic in the knowledge that she had gathered these blossoms, then silently entered the bedroom to leave them for his eyes alone. Was the nosegay a comment on what had happened earlier? A thank-you for Moonbeam? Or some other, subtler message?

He placed the flowers in a glass of water and set it on his bedside table. Yet as he turned off the lamp, he had the nagging feeling that there was something he was missing about the nosegay. Perhaps he'd think of it in the morning.

Instead he fell asleep, and dreamed of his brother.

Shouts of laughter as he and Kyle played with conkers as boys. Sneaking out of the house when they were supposed to be studying so they could attend a forbidden village fair. Waking in the middle of the night knowing that Kyle was hurt, and finding him with an injured ankle after falling down the steps on a midnight pantry raid.

And darker times. Fighting with fists, and with words that hurt more than blows. Kyle's increased arrogance when he returned from his first term at Eton with the apparent belief that Dominic should be a follower rather than an equal. The steely, glinting fury in Kyle's eyes whenever Dominic took independent action. Competing for the favors of a barmaid, and the blaze of satisfaction when she preferred him to Viscount Maxwell.

The last, devastating battle when Dominic chose the army over the university...

During the Christmas holidays of Dominic's last year at Rugby, he was summoned to his father's study and told it was time to decide his future. Dominic knew that the choices for a younger son were the church and the army. The trouble was that he wanted neither of those. His real desire was to manage an estate, preferably his own, though he'd work for someone else if necessary. If he earned a decent salary and saved most of his allowance, eventually he'd be able to buy a farm.

Timidly he'd asked if he could train as a steward, perhaps at a smaller family property rather than Dornleigh. The suggestion had been brusquely refused; a Renbourne would not become a hireling. The earl said that he would pay for a university education if Dominic chose to become a vicar, or buy a commission in a suitable regiment if that was his son's choice. Dominic had until the end of the holidays to decide.

Even though Kyle was also home and the two of them were rubbing along tolerably well, instinctively Dominic kept the matter of his future to himself, knowing that his brother would try to influence his decision. For days he went back and forth. He'd rather enjoyed his studies at Rugby and done quite well with them. He'd probably enjoy three years at a university, too. But—a vicar? On the other hand, he didn't feel any great calling to be a soldier, either.

The night before returning to school, he made up his mind as he and his brother were shooting billiards after dinner. Kyle was lining up a shot when Dominic announced, "I'm going into the army. A cavalry regiment, I think." He smiled, as if the decision had been easy. "Shall I become a hussar? They have the most dashing uniforms."

His brother's cue stick jerked and the shot went wild. Kyle straightened, his face pale. "You can't be serious. You just said that to ruin my shot, didn't you?"

Dominic took his turn and neatly potted a ball. "I have to do something, and the army seems the best choice. I shouldn't think I'd like the navy."

"I thought you'd come to Cambridge with me." Kyle slid his cue stick restlessly between his hands. "We could share a set of rooms. It...it would be like old times."

Old times. The thought was tempting. Dominic made another shot as he considered, then reluctantly shook his head. "If you can see me as a vicar, your imagination is better than mine."

"You'd make a perfectly decent cleric," Kyle said seriously. "You're patient and good with people. The living here at Dornleigh should be available in five years or so, when old Simpson retires. That would be perfect. The income is good, and I'm sure that Wrexham would be happy to give you the living when you're ready."

Dominic shuddered at the thought. To spend the rest of his life within a mile of the family seat while living as a poor relation? He didn't know much about heaven, but he was quite sure that being vicar of Dornleigh would be hell. Cutting off his brother's enthusiasm, he said, "It wouldn't work, Kyle. I'd be bored to tears. At least in the cavalry, there might be some excitement now and then."

"For God's sake, Dom! Only a damned fool would join the army," Kyle snapped.

Dominic would have laughed if anyone else had said that, but only his brother could anger him thus. "Your opinion is so flattering." Eyes narrowed, he bent over the table and grimly scored one ball after another, ending the game. "I may be a damned fool, but I can still beat you at billiards, or anything else."

"Damnation, Dom!" Kyle glared across the table. "This is your life we're talking about, not a blasted game. You've got a brain. Use it! Come to Cambridge. If you don't want the church, read law. You'd be good at that, too. But for heaven's sake, don't waste yourself as cannon fodder."

A lifetime locked in dusty rooms with dusty books...did Kyle know so little of his brother? Did he care about nothing but indulging his desire for a companion at Cambridge? "There are many who think defending one's country is an honorable calling. And even if it weren't, being ten minutes older gives you no right to dictate how I should spend my life."

"Is that what you think I'm trying to do?" Kyle took a deep breath, visibly struggling with his temper. "I want what's best for you. With Napoleon exiled in Elba, you'll be as bored in the army as you would be in the vicarage. Continue your education instead. Three years from now, you might feel differently about what you want to do." His voice softened. "Please, Dom. I'd like to have you there."

The appeal affected Dominic far more than Kyle's anger had. Maybe his brother had a point. No one was a better companion than Kyle in a good mood. It would be like when they were boys...

But they were no longer boys, and the pleasant vision was shattered by the sudden knowledge that falling in with his brother's plans would be spiritual suicide. Whenever they were together, Kyle was the Heir and Dominic was the Spare. He would slowly fade into the shadows, of no importance to himself or anyone.

If he was ever to be his own man, he had to leave. "That wouldn't do, Kyle," he said with finality. "The army will suit me well enough. If the rumors come true and Napoleon leaves Elba, I might even be useful."

"No!" Kyle smashed his cue stick violently across the edge of the billiard table, splintering it into shards. For a moment it seemed as if he would hurl himself across the table and lock his hands around his brother's throat. Instead, he said with lethal intensity, "If you do this, I swear before God that I will never forgive you."

Dominic felt the blood drain from his face. "How fortunate that I have no interest in your forgiveness." Then he spun on his heel and left the room.

He'd been proud of the fact that he didn't start to shake until he reached the privacy of his own bedroom.

Dominic wakened from the dream, still hearing his twin's voice ringing in his ears. As he stared into the darkness, he knew he'd made the right decision. Yet now, a decade later, he saw with crystal clarity that Kyle's bullying had been rooted as much in concern as in the desire to impose his will. A pity that Dominic hadn't understood then, because his anger with his brother had deepened the schism.

After Waterloo he'd yearned to return home and spend time with Kyle. Perhaps a trip into Scotland, where they could ride and fish and hike through familiar green hills. Some evening, after a generous amount of brandy, Dominic would have spoken of the hell of battle. Though Kyle wouldn't have said much—men didn't talk about such things—his quiet understanding would have healed invisible wounds.

But Dominic could no longer turn to his brother. Though the companionship of his fellow officers had saved him from total breakdown, it had not been the same. The scars of holding the pain inside were with him still. He'd spoken to no one until today, when he'd told Meriel.

Odd how close he felt to her, despite her mental quirks. Thinking of that closeness brought back the memory of the kiss they had shared, a topic so alarming that it was a relief when his restless mind circled back to his brother.

Despite their estrangement, there was still a connection between them. Several years earlier, Dominic had been thrown while hunting in the Shires. His horse had to be destroyed, while he'd suffered broken bones and a cracked skull. Kyle arrived from London the next evening, growling and scolding his brother for riding like a ham-handed peasant. If Dominic had felt less wretched, he would have hit Kyle. Instead, though he would never have admitted it aloud, he'd been embarrassingly glad to see him.

Kyle had finished his waspish lecture by dismissing the local sawbones hired by Dominic's hunting friends. Then he'd summoned the best physician in the Midlands. Dominic's next memories were hazy, dreamlike images of Kyle sitting with him all night when he was half out of his mind with fever. His brother had sponged his face with cool water, and pressed him back to the bed when he tried to flounder up.

After the fever broke, Dominic decided he'd dreamed those scenes, because Kyle had shown no disposition to play nursemaid. He'd barely even been civil.

As soon as Dominic was on the road to recovery, Kyle had left without explaining how he'd learned of the accident so quickly. Only later did Dominic discover that none of his friends had thought to notify the Renbourne family of his injury; the mysterious bond forged when they were boys was what brought Kyle to his side. His brother had known of his injury at Waterloo, too, though Dominic hadn't learned that until much later. As a boy, such sensations had been routine; sometimes he hadn't known whether he was experiencing his own emotions, or Kyle's. He'd deliberately suppressed such feelings after their estrangement, with only partial success.

His throat tightened with sorrow. How had he and his brother come to such a pass? Surely they could have done better. If Kyle had been less imperious. If Dominic had been more patient instead of allowing his brother to goad him into anger.

The past couldn't be changed, but perhaps the future could be. Silently he vowed to hold on to his temper the next time they met, and to avoid saying things he knew would provoke his twin. And for God's sake, he absolutely must not behave improperly to his brother's bride. One didn't have to be twin-born to know that Kyle would find that unforgivable. He would assume that Dominic was deliberately trifling with Meriel as part of their lifelong competition.

When was the last time they were really close? Probably it had been when their mother died. The countess had been stricken with a sudden fever, and both boys had been summoned home from school. Rugby was closer, and Dominic had reached Dornleigh first. She'd smiled and whispered his name, for she had never once confused her two sons. Voice barely audible, she added, "Look out for your brother. He isn't like you. He...breaks more easily."

Soon after that, she'd slipped into a sleep from which she never woke. His face like granite, the earl withdrew to his study. Dominic watched for his brother's carriage, aching, and thought of what his mother had said. Silently he vowed not to repeat her exact words, for Kyle would be humiliated to think that she'd considered him weak. Dominic knew that wasn't what she meant, but it was better not to try to explain.

Kyle arrived home late that night. Dominic raced down the stairs to the front hall, knowing that he should be the one to break the news. As soon as Kyle entered, his gaze went to his twin, pleading wordlessly for hope.

Dominic shook his head, throat tight. "She's gone, Kyle. The...the last thing she did was speak of you. She sent her love." For that, after all, was what her words had really meant.

Kyle's expression shattered. "She died and I wasn't here. *I wasn't here!*"

Undone by Kyle's anguish, Dominic reached out to his brother. They ended up clinging together as Kyle sobbed uncontrollably. Tears ran down his own cheeks, and they were united in grief as they never were again.

The memory of that grief resonated strangely. Dominic gradually realized that he could feel his brother now. And tonight he sensed the same terrible grief he'd felt the day Kyle had asked him to come to Warfield. In fact, the sorrow seemed even deeper now. What the devil was going on?

Another thought struck with the force of absolute conviction. Kyle was out of the country. Ireland? No, farther than that. France, perhaps, or maybe even Spain or Portugal. No wonder he'd said that no messages could reach him. But why go abroad now? If this was a simple pleasure trip, he surely could have postponed it. Nor would there be such sorrow emanating from him that Dominic could feel it hundreds of miles away. Damnation, but he wished there was something he could do.

Perhaps there was. If he could feel Kyle, perhaps his brother could feel him.

He tried to formulate a prayer but swiftly gave that up. He had no gift for holy words. Instead, he imagined himself reaching out, through the night and the uncounted miles, and laying his hand on his brother's shoulder. Letting him know that he was not alone, despite the physical and emotional distance that separated them. Perhaps it was his imagination, but he thought he sensed an easing of Kyle's grief. He hoped so.

Exhausted by the turbulent day, he rolled

on his side and attempted sleep again. But his mind still churned with thoughts of Kyle, and of Meriel. His future sister-in-law.

He *must* not allow his relationship with her to become any closer. Already he was on dangerous ground. The potential conflict with his brother was the catastrophic kind that ripped families apart forever.

Yet surely it would not hurt to take the nosegay Meriel had made and inhale the fragrance once more. Spice and sweetness, just like her.

Flowers curled in his hand, he finally drifted into sleep.

Chapter 18

"You have a visitor, my lord."

Dominic glanced up from where he was laboriously transplanting small cabbages so they could grow into large cabbages. The young housemaid who had delivered the message promptly blushed, overcome by the enormity of talking to him.

Who the devil would be calling on him at Warfield? He got to his feet, ruefully noting the muddy stains on his knees. Rain in the night was good for the garden but messy for the gardeners. "Who is it?"

The housemaid looked stricken. "I...I forgot, my lord. Nor did she have a card. A proper lady, though."

Probably some distant Renbourne relative who lived in the area and had heard that Lord Maxwell was visiting Warfield. Well, whoever it was would have to accept him in all his muddy glory. He called, "Kamal, I have a visitor. I'll be back soon."

The Indian looked up from the bed he was hoeing. "Very good, my lord."

Meriel, who was thinning the blossoms on pepper bushes so they would bear larger fruit later, continued to softly croon one of her wordless melodies, but she gave Dominic a swift, unreadable glance. In the three days since he'd visited the asylum and given her Moonbeam, they had not been alone together.

Perhaps it was coincidence that all her projects had involved working with Kamal, but Dominic doubted it. Clearly she wanted chaperoning. Very wise of her. But he missed the easy companionship of the two of them gardening alone. Though he liked Kamal, having him around all the time changed things.

Dominic followed the maid back to the house, pausing only long enough to wash his hands at the glasshouse. Changing his clothes would waste another half hour, and he'd just get muddy again when he returned to the kitchen garden.

The visitor was sharing a tea tray with the ladies in the small parlor. His entrance interrupted a buzz of conversation, and three sets of female eyes turned toward him. The visitor, an attractive, fashionable woman around his age, looked vaguely familiar, but he couldn't place her. Lord, he hoped she wasn't some former mistress of his brother's!

Using Kyle's most smoothly arrogant tone, the one that said Lord Maxwell was always correctly attired, even when he looked as if he'd been dragged through a bush backward, Dominic said, "Pray forgive my appearance. I thought the rudeness of coming to you direct from the garden to be less than the rudeness of making you wait."

The visitor rose to her feet. Tall and imposing, she had short dark hair and dramatic brown eyes. "I would be the last person on earth to criticize you, Lord Maxwell. I am too much in your debt."

He studied her face. They'd met, and not that long ago, but when?

She smiled a little. "You don't recognize me. I'm glad."

Her voice triggered the memory. But then she had been screaming, on the verge of hysteria. "Gods above," he said blankly. "Mrs. Morton." He bowed over her gloved hand, amazed and delighted at how her appearance had changed since the asylum.

"I am Jena Ames once more." Her expression hardened. "I shall never use that man's name again."

"One can hardly blame you, my dear." Mrs. Marks poured a fresh cup of tea. "Miss Ames has been telling us about her husband's wickedness, and how she is free today because of your actions. You are a hero, my lord."

He made a dismissive gesture with his hand,

ashamed to think how close he had come to not bothering. "All I did was carry a message."

"Nonetheless, I am here to thank you," Jena said quietly. "If you had not listened to a woman presumed mad, I doubt I would ever have been freed from the asylum. My keepers would not have allowed me another chance to distress a visitor."

Accepting a cup of tea, he settled into a wooden chair, not wanting to soil upholstery. His gaze went over Jena Ames again. She was the image of a confident woman, sure of herself and her place in the world. Only the shadows under her eyes revealed how much she had recently suffered.

Still, as the conversation continued, he began to notice signs of increasing tension. When he'd finished his tea, he suggested, "Since Miss Ames knew Meriel in India, perhaps she'd like to go outside and see her today."

Jena hesitated. "If...if you think she wouldn't mind."

"I'm sure she wouldn't." He rose from his seat and glanced at the ladies. "Would you like to stroll out to the kitchen garden with us?"

As he'd hoped, Mrs. Marks said, "Too hot. You young people run along."

He offered his arm to Jena. Again she hesitated, as if uncertain, before taking it. Together they exited from the back of the house into the parterre. She released her breath in a long sigh. "The fresh air feels so *good*, Lord Maxwell. So...so free."

Thinking this would be a good chance to learn about Meriel's earlier years, he said, "Since it's a fine day, would you like to take an indirect route to our destination?"

"Please." She gave him a sidelong glance. "You saw that I was becoming rather frayed, didn't you?"

"I thought that might be happening," he admitted. "After your ordeal in the asylum, it must be something of a strain to reenter society."

"I'm afraid so, even though Mrs. Marks and Mrs. Rector could not have been kinder." She gave him a rueful smile. "I feel as if I'm walking on eggs. My father pushed me out the door today, saying that the sooner I resume normal life, the better. I know he is right, but I feel rather like an ensign being sent off into battle."

It was an example he could understand. "A general must be a good judge of people, I think. Your father wouldn't ask more than you can manage."

Her smile became genuine. "He is the best of fathers. I should have listened when he told me that Morton was a fortune hunter, but I didn't want to believe him."

Dominic wondered what would become of her husband, but didn't ask. With the general taking care of his daughter's interests, Morton would get what he deserved.

They turned down a long walk that ran between banks of assorted flowers. Enormous effort had gone into making the rich tangle of blossoms appear natural. At the end of the walk stood an ancient statue of Artemis, the moon goddess. Her slim, half-wild figure reminded him of Meriel. "What was Meriel like as a child?"

"Bright and sweet and ethereal. She looked up to me, since I was several years older." Jena laughed. "I enjoyed having a disciple. We were inseparable during the month she and her parents stayed at Cambay. She was small for her age, but clever as a whip. Did you know that she'd learned to read when she was only four years old? What happened to her was such a terrible, terrible waste."

He felt a deep pang, wondering what Meriel might be now if her parents had chosen a different route through India. "You never saw her again after that visit?"

Jena's face clouded. "Actually, the maharajah sent her to Cambay, since it was the nearest British cantonment. She was recognized immediately, of course. That's how she was returned to her family."

"I've wondered how an Indian prince explained having a captive English child," Dominic said. "Do you know the story?"

"He said she'd been one of a number of gifts presented to him by a neighboring ruler. She was thought to be a Circassian slave because of her coloring, and since she never spoke, no one was the wiser. Eventually the maharani decided she must be English, so they sent her to Cambay." Jena shrugged. "She was fortunate. A maharajah's zenana is large enough for a small child to be overlooked indefinitely."

They had reached the statue of Artemis. He looked up into the blank, otherworldly stone eyes. "Did you see Meriel while she stayed in Cambay?"

"I was told that she was unwell, but I demanded to be allowed to visit her. I thought perhaps I could reach her when the doctors couldn't. She stared right through me. It was the uncanniest thing. As if I was a ghost. Or she was." Jena's mouth twisted. "I was furious, as if she'd deliberately turned away from our friendship."

"You were still a child yourself," he said mildly. "It's understandable that you were upset that she had changed so much."

Jena studied his face. "You are a very restful man, Lord Maxwell. Easy to talk to. I should think you are very good for Meriel."

He blinked, startled. He would have said it was the other way around. Being around Meriel made him happier and more focused than he'd been in at least a decade. She could be a maddening little sprite, but the world was a more interesting place for her presence. Reminding himself acerbically that he was not supposed to think of her with such fondness, he said simply, "I like her, and hope she likes me."

Leaving Artemis, he guided Jena into a fragrance garden that had been planted to release a succession of scents throughout the year. At the moment, the headiness of lilac dominated. "Did you call on Meriel when you returned to England?"

"I considered it, but didn't. It's common knowledge in Shropshire that Lady Meriel is mad." Jena smiled self-mockingly. "I told myself that I didn't want to upset her, but the truth is that I didn't want to be disturbed myself. The thought of her madness repelled me. I've been royally punished for my lack of compassion."

"Perhaps the time was not right to call on her," he said thoughtfully. "Now you have much more understanding of mental disorders."

"That's certainly true. Sometimes I wondered if I was going mad myself." Jena's face tightened. "I can understand now why Meriel drew into herself—it was a way of surviving an intolerable world. I raged when I was first confined at Bladenham, and spent quite a bit of time in restraints. But as hopelessness set in, I found myself withdrawing more and more. There were days when I simply lay on my cot and stared at the ceiling, ignoring the attendants as if that would make them vanish."

"What would bring you back to the world again?"

She thought about it. "Boredom or physical restlessness, I suppose. Or necessity. When you came to Bladenham I was taking my outdoor exercise as mindless as a honeybee, until I realized there was an outsider close enough to talk to. It was like a splash of ice water, because I hadn't seen another person from outside the asylum the whole time I was at

Bladenham. I knew I might never have such a chance again, so I watched like a hawk for the best time to approach you."

He nodded. The women's situations were very different, since Jena had never really been mad, only worn down by misery and despair. Meriel had been far more deeply damaged, and at a very tender age.

"What is Meriel like now?" Jena asked. "Is there anything I should know?"

"She doesn't speak, and is still quite capable of ignoring people." He gestured at their surroundings. "She spends most of her time working in the gardens, and does it very well. I think she has been opening up to the world a bit more, but I suppose I haven't known her long enough to be sure. I shall let you draw your own conclusions."

A few more minutes of walking brought them to the kitchen garden. The sky had clouded up, so Meriel had discarded her hat. Her flaxen braid fell over her shoulder as she leaned forward to attend to her pepper plants.

Jena said quietly, "I would have recognized her anywhere. She looks...serene."

"Most of the time, she is. This is her home."

"And infinitely better than any asylum." Jena scanned the kitchen garden, her brows drawing together when she saw Kamal. "The Indian—he looks familiar."

"You might have seen Kamal at Cambay. He escorted Meriel from the maharajah's palace," Dominic explained. "He's been with her ever since."

After a last, intent look at the Indian, Jena took a deep breath and stepped forward. "Hello, Meriel. Do you remember me after all these years?" Heedless of the damp ground, she knelt beside Meriel. "I'm Jena Ames. From Cambay."

Meriel stiffened and kept her head down, pointedly ignoring her visitor. Undeterred, Jena said softly, "We were such good friends then. Do you remember how we used to ride together? How much you loved the Indian gardens I showed you? Before leaving Cambay, you gave me your favorite doll so I would remember you. In return, I gave you a small book of poems I had copied by hand. We...we promised to visit again someday, when I came back to England." Tears glinted in Jena's eyes, but didn't fall. "Here I am, Meriel. It's taken a long time, but I never forgot you."

In the silence that followed, only the hum of bees could be heard. On the other side of the kitchen garden, Kamal had stopped and was watching as intently as Dominic.

Meriel pinched off a pepper blossom. Then, jerkily, she raised her head and looked Jena in the face. Their gazes locked.

Dominic held his breath as he watched, half expecting them to touch noses, like two cats meeting for the first time. Slowly Meriel lifted her hand and touched Jena's cheek. Then she smiled with swift radiance.

Jena caught Meriel's hand, her face lighting up. "It's so good to see you again!"

Dominic exhaled with relief. His gaze went

to Kamal, who gave a faint nod. It mattered that Meriel had recognized someone from her past.

Meriel's tunic sleeves were rolled up, revealing a bracelet pattern on her right wrist. Jena's gaze fell on it. "A mehndi! You were fascinated by them. Remember how I had our housekeeper paint mehndi on our hands? You asked questions the whole time." Glancing at Kamal, she asked something in a foreign language.

He shook his head and replied in English. "No, memsahib. I obtain the henna and taught Meriel how to use it, but she is the artist."

Jena looked at Meriel again. "Would you do mehndi for me? It would be like old times." There was a wistful note in her voice for the lost innocence of two little girls who had been friends when life was simple.

Meriel rose gracefully and snapped her fingers for Roxana, who sprawled nearby. Then she collected Jena with a glance, and they all headed toward the house.

Feeling almost giddy, Dominic crossed the garden to Kamal. "Meriel understood Jena's question, and is responding to it! She really is getting better—it's not just my imagination."

"Your presence is good for her." Kamal deftly chopped a weed from the soil with his sharp-edged hoe. "You bear a great responsibility. When teaching a young bird to fly, one must not let it fall."

Dominic sobered. "I don't intend to let her fall."

"No?" Kamal's gaze was so piercing that

Dominic wondered uneasily if the Indian suspected that he was not Lord Maxwell. But Kamal said no more. Looking down, he neatly removed a tangled clump of weeds.

Dominic returned to the work of transplanting cabbages, his mood troubled. He'd thought in terms of helping Meriel to move into the outside world. Once she had mastered a larger life, she would not need his help. But what if she expected regular attention from her husband? Would Kyle provide that?

He imagined Kyle with Meriel, and his fingers tightened, snapping a fragile seedling. How could any man not want to be with Meriel as much as possible?

Chapter 19

*I*ndia. *Arms locked around her knees, Meriel sat on the window seat of her darkened bedroom, rocking slightly. Seeing Jena had released a torrent of distant memories that seemed almost to belong to a stranger. For years she'd refused to think of India, though nightmare fragments of horror and fire haunted her dreams.*

But now the vivid colors and scents of the subcontinent threatened to overwhelm her. The first months had been a grand adventure of exotic plants, beasts, and people, completely different from Warfield. But there had been few playmates, until she met Jena. Despite their differences there had been an affinity, a sense that each had found the sister she'd always wanted. The month at Cambay had been perhaps the happiest of her life, for she'd had excitement, her parents, and her friend.

Then they left the cantonment—how long? she could no longer remember—and the secure life she had known shattered when the cruelty beneath India's beauty erupted into death and destruction. She'd survived by escaping in her mind, going back to the cool green hills of home.

Warfield became more real than the madness around her. The best day of her life had been when her uncle had brought her back. Her land had been the one constant of her existence, the truest and the safest thing in her life. She wanted no one and nothing more.

At least, that was all she had wanted until Renbourne came, with his probing gaze and dangerous allure.

Now Jena had arrived to roil the waters still more. While Meriel painted mehndi, her old friend had spoken haltingly of her husband's betrayal and the horrible months in the asylum. Her dark eyes had been haunted by sadness, yet her essential spirit was undimmed. She'd always been a creature of fire, forceful and impetuous, and her presence brought back so much. Too much. Meriel thought sorrowfully of the doll she had given Jena, and the book of painstakingly copied poems she had received in return, now long gone to ash.

Rocking harder, she buried her face against her knees.

Dominic sighed as he took off his coat and loosened his cravat. Meriel had skipped dinner again. Sometimes he wondered if his presence was driving her to starvation. She must live on sunshine and spring rain, like a flower.

According to the ladies, Jena Ames had left smiling, her wrists decorated with mehndi, and promising to call again soon. Meriel had apparently enjoyed the encounter, but she'd vanished by the time Dominic came inside at the end of the afternoon. During dinner and a friendly game of cards he'd hoped she would appear. No such luck.

He pulled back the coverlet on his bed and found another nosegay between the pillows. A small bundle of pinks, tied with a strand of white yarn. Meriel might have missed dinner, but she'd been here. The thought quickened his pulse as he inhaled the spicy scent of the flowers. Why had she left them?

The language of flowers! There was a whole system of flower symbolism, just as there was a language of fan gestures. He didn't know the exact meanings, but it was a fair guess that Meriel's nosegays were meant to tease and captivate. Very successful, too.

After a day of vigorous physical work he should have been ready for bed, but he wasn't. His mind was buzzing too much to allow sleep anytime soon. On impulse, he decided to go down to the library and look for books on India, since that was where Meriel's life had taken its tragic turn. Learning more about what

212

she must have experienced might increase his understanding of her.

Kyle knew about India; he'd always loved reading books about exotic lands. Dominic wondered if his brother had yet traveled the five hundred miles from London necessary to qualify for the Travellers Club. Wrexham kept his heir on a short leash.

Not sure whether he was glad or irritated that Kyle would certainly be well informed about the country where his bride had lived for two critical years, Dominic took a lamp and silently went downstairs. The library was an appealing place, well stocked with books and comfortable furniture. He'd like to see it on a cold rainy day, with fires burning in the two fireplaces and Meriel and her pets for company.

The door was open when he reached it, with light visible inside. One of the ladies must be looking for late night reading, too. He paused in the doorway, his gaze scanning the room. A branch of candles was lit at the far end. At the edge of the circle of light, a small feminine figure stood beside a bookshelf, engrossed in a volume in her hands. The lack of height and the silvery hair made him assume it was Mrs. Rector.

Then she shelved the book and pulled down another, turning so that he could see her more clearly. His jaw dropped. Meriel. And she was *reading*! The shock was as great as when he'd heard her sing and realized that she wasn't mute.

Could she be merely looking at engravings in an illustrated volume? He watched as her eyes scanned back and forth. Definitely reading. Jena Ames had said Meriel had learned to read at age four, but he'd assumed that she lost that skill along with so many others after the trauma of her abduction. Instead, she had secretly continued to read.

On the verge of explosion, he stalked into the library. Meriel's head whipped up when she heard his footsteps. She froze, her eyes narrow and feline.

"What a surprise, Lady Meriel," he said icily. "What kind of book catches your fancy?"

Her eyes flickered as she considered flight, but she would never be able to get by him to a door. Halting in front of her, he plucked the volume from her hands. "William Blake, *Songs of Innocence*." A poet and artist widely considered to be mad, though Dominic rather enjoyed his work. His otherworldly writing and illustrations must suit Meriel admirably.

He set the book on the table and picked up another slim volume. John Keats. He flipped it open, and his eyes fell on a verse.

> *I met a lady in the meads*
> *Full beautiful, a faery's child;*
> *Her hair was long, her foot was light,*
> *And her eyes were wild.*

He slammed the book shut. Sweet Jesus! Keats couldn't have met Meriel before writing "La Belle Dame Sans Merci," but he'd described her to perfection.

Struggling to keep his temper and sense of

hurt under control, he said, "So you've been playing us all for fools. If you can read, you can certainly understand spoken language. You know everything that's going on around you. This whole great household revolves around your whims and needs, with everyone trying to please you. You accept it all, and give back nothing. *Nothing!*"

When his voice rose, she bolted, darting around him toward the door. He caught her shoulders and swung her around, then had to dodge her clawing hands. "Behave yourself, you little wildcat!"

He yanked off his loose cravat and swiftly tied her wrists together. She kicked him, but bare feet couldn't do much damage. Sweeping her up in his arms, he carried her to a wing chair where the candlelight would fall full on her face.

He deposited her none too gently, then pulled another chair opposite hers and sat down so closely that their knees almost touched. In her eyes he saw glints of rage and resentment, but of madness there was none.

More quietly, he asked, "Why, Meriel? If you can sing and read, you're capable of talking if you want. I'm sure of it. Why have you kept silent for so many years?"

Her head turned sharply so he could no longer see into her eyes. She gave up trying to escape and drew herself into a tight ball, rejecting him and everything around her. Wearing a silk dressing gown belted over a fine lawn night robe, she looked small and delicate and feminine.

Feeling like a brute, he untied her bound hands and tossed his cravat aside. "Running is your method of avoiding hard questions, isn't it? You have everyone so convinced that you're witless that you can get away with anything you want. It's freedom of sorts, but you're paying a damnably high price."

Still no response, though he didn't doubt that she understood every word he'd said. A swift pulse hammered in her throat. Brain and tongue might be capable of speech, but she wasn't going to offer any.

Frustrated, he took a deep breath and tried to imagine himself in her place. A bright, sensitive, protected child who was brutally torn from her family and her familiar world, she had withdrawn from harsh reality to survive. For a year or more, she'd not had anyone to speak with even if she'd wanted that. He could understand why terror and misery had traumatized her into silence. But why didn't she eventually regain her speech, after she was restored to the keeping of people who loved her?

Because once she began to speak, she would never be able to return to her private world. "Silence is your shield, isn't it?" he said slowly. "To converse with others would mean irrevocably stepping into the normal world. As a child, you would have had to answer painful questions about how your parents died, and what happened to you in captivity. As you became older, normalcy would mean obligations. Responsibilities. You would have been packed off to London to find a husband, for example."

She shuddered and bit her lip.

Her response triggered another insight. "The Marriage Mart is enough to unnerve anyone, but for you the real horror would be leaving your home, I think." He remembered her reaction to going outside the wall. "It was a terrible strain for you to travel even a mile outside Warfield Park. If you were a 'normal' young lady, you would be expected to do far more than that."

She sighed, her lids dropping for an instant. Even if he was right—and he was sure he was—she wasn't ready to admit it.

He leaned forward earnestly. "Will you talk to me, Meriel? If you wish, I'll swear to tell no one else. But I'd like so much to hear you speak." Her voice would be light and musical, he thought. Like fairy bells.

"You may have found safety in silence, but you're missing so much. Good conversation is one of life's great pleasures." He thought with a pang of the endless discussions between him and Kyle in the days when they were friends. Their thoughts had completed and enhanced one another, sparking new ideas. "Sharing thoughts aloud is the closest two people can come without touching physically. In fact, speech is often far more intimate than touch."

Indecision showed on her expressive face. He held his breath, sensing that she was on the verge of abandoning the defenses that had become part of her. He also realized wryly that his last statement had been less than the truth. Though she had never spoken a word to him, he felt achingly close to her.

Her expression changed as she made up her mind, but instead of speaking, she straightened her knotted body. Then, slowly, sinuously, she placed her feet on the floor and stood, her bare toes almost touching his shoes and her gaze holding his. It was a novel sensation to look up at her.

She was indecently close, so he pushed himself back in his chair as he wondered what the devil she had in mind. He no longer believed she was mad—but neither was she like anyone else.

Eyes gazing deep into his, she untied the ribbon that secured her braid. Then she combed her fingers through her heavy flaxen hair until it loosened into a shining, rosemary-scented cascade that spilled past her waist.

His nails dug into the arms of his chair as he fought the temptation to reach out and touch. Women had been made queens and empires had fallen because of such magnificent hair. Throat dry, he said, "If you're trying to distract me, it won't work. You are...very lovely, but I'd rather hear you talk, even if only to curse me."

Holding his gaze, she unbelted her robe. A shimmy of her shoulders sent it sliding down her arms and onto the floor. The lawn nightgown beneath was exquisitely embroidered, befitting an heiress, and her narrow wrists emerged from falls of creamy lace. He stared at the translucent fabric, which revealed tantalizing hints of her slim body. Gods above, he should run fast and far, but he could not even force himself to turn his eyes away from the mesmerizing sight.

She bent her head and pressed her lips to his temple. Her hair swept silkily forward over his face, erotic beyond words as she nibbled across his cheek with butterfly lightness. Heart hammering, he reached up and cupped her face between his hands, drawing her into a kiss. Her mouth opened with welcome, warm and intoxicating.

As the kiss went on and on, she flowed into his lap, straddling him. Lithe and willing, she was the stuff of dreams and madness.

This was madness. Gasping for air and sanity, he set her back a little, saying unsteadily, "You're really, really good at changing the subject, little witch."

She laughed softly and buried her face against his throat, inhaling his scent as her tongue trailed teasingly toward his ear. At the same time, she curled her hips against his, bracketing his groin with intimate heat.

Sense shattered. Yearning to possess her, to become inextricably twined in body and soul, he caught her in his arms and laid her down on the thick Persian carpet, an ivory princess framed in voluptuous crimson. His devouring mouth traveled from soft lips to smooth throat, then to the curves provocatively covered by her sheer nightgown. Her breast was small and perfectly formed, like the rest of her, and her nipple hardened against his tongue.

She gasped, and one of her hands circled his neck as her other arm locked around his back. As he reached for the hem of her robe, she laughed with rich feminine triumph.

A fragment of sanity fought through his mind. He no longer believed her incapable of understanding her own actions. She knew exactly what she was about, even if her understanding came from Mother Eve rather than English society. She was discovering her female power—but it would do neither of them any good if she persuaded him to abandon morals and honor for a swift, disastrous rush of passion.

Panting, he pushed himself up so that he was braced above her. She was a portrait of wanton innocence, her eyes clouded with desire. Her lips curved into an intimate smile, and he wanted nothing more than to kiss her again.

Instead, he said shakily, "You may be a pagan by preference, but you surely know that society condemns coupling outside of marriage."

Her expression changed. Confused, she reached for him, one hand running down his body. He rolled out of touching distance and fought to cool his raging blood. "Would you talk if that would persuade me to become your lover?" he said, his voice edged. "Or is seduction your way of avoiding my questions?"

Her eyes widened with outrage. With one swift move, she pulled herself into a crouch, hissing like a cat. He guessed that she was very close to clawing at him. It would almost be funny, if the situation weren't so wrenching.

"I know you're angry. I'm not very happy myself," he said quietly. "But I swear that I want what is best for you, Meriel. You're like a princess in a tower, high above the hurly-burly of daily life. No doubt you feel very safe and superior up there, but a tower is a lonely place if you won't let anyone in."

He caught her tense hand, hoping the warmth of his clasp would soften it. "I want rather desperately for you to let me in. But our minds must meet before our bodies can."

Her lips parted, and for a suspended instant he thought she was on the verge of speech. Then she yanked her hand free and sprang to her feet, scooping up her robe as she did. Back erect, she stalked from the library like an offended lioness.

This time, he let her go.

Mind and body seething, he let himself out into the moonlit night and made his way toward the old castle with long, desperate strides. What was madness, what was sanity? He was half mad himself right now. More than half mad, to have allowed that scene. If Meriel had accepted his challenge to speak, would he have been honor-bound to make love to her? Would he have been capable of stopping himself from doing so? No wonder society hedged a young girl's virtue with so many protections. Without those rules, it was catastrophically easy for passion to overrule sense.

God knew that he was living proof of that, for despite all his warnings to himself, he had fallen in love with her. She elicited tenderness and desire, laughter and wonder, a fierce need to protect her from all threats.

With the cool clarity of hindsight, he saw how severing his ties with his family to become his own man had been only the first step. Yes, he'd saved himself from becoming his brother's shadow, but he hadn't taken the next step into maturity. Instead he had drifted aimlessly for years because his most powerful desire— to sink his roots deep into his own land— seemed unattainable. That was why he'd jumped at Kyle's offer of Bradshaw Manor, even though it meant becoming a liar. To be a landowner would give his life purpose.

Now Meriel had given him an even greater sense of purpose, for what higher goal could a man have than to protect and serve those he loved?

As he climbed the path to the castle ruins, a treacherous idea insinuated itself into his mind. What if he asked Meriel to marry *him*, Dominic Renbourne, not the absent lord who was her intended? Amworth wanted a loving husband who would treat Meriel well, and Dominic was the best possible choice, for no one else could love her more.

But how could he support her? His younger

son's allowance was only enough for a bachelor.

Then he remembered, with a cold, sick twist in the belly, that she was a great heiress. Meriel didn't need his support—on the contrary, her fortune could support them in luxury for the rest of their lives. The world—including Amworth—would think him an opportunist, a fortune hunter who had seduced his brother's hapless bride. *Christ.*

Did he care what the world thought? In this, yes. He'd never much minded being considered a wastrel, but the idea that people would believe he'd taken advantage of a vulnerable innocent revolted him.

But even that was not as bad as the prospect of Kyle's reaction. His brother hadn't had the chance to fall in love with Meriel, but he must have been dazzled by her beauty. Certainly he was set upon this marriage. For Dominic to steal her away would be an unforgivable betrayal.

As Dominic entered the moonlight-drenched precincts of the castle, he grimly faced the fact that for him to wed Meriel would destroy anything that remained of the bond that had been formed between Kyle and him in the womb. Lord Maxwell was untrusting to begin with—too many people wanted things from a future earl. If Dominic betrayed his brother in such a fundamental way, he would cause irrevocable damage.

Slowly he climbed the stone steps to the battlements, thinking of his first visit. Meriel had frightened him half to death when she had stepped off the wall. That was the day he had begun to fall in love with her, for he had seen first her diabolical humor and then her compassion, when she had attacked a poacher twice her size in defense of a wounded fox.

The memory of her going after the poacher twisted his heart with longing. She was so gallant. So rare.

The sobering truth was that he was already so deeply involved with Meriel that to withdraw would be a betrayal as profound as what he would do to Kyle if he claimed his brother's bride for his own. How the *hell* could he have been so stupid—so crazy—as to allow this to happen?

Leaning on the battlements, he looked over the wall to the dark, moon-silvered river far below. Easy to understand how someone in distress could be lured into jumping. A few instants of flight, and then oblivion. Deliverance from an impossible dilemma.

Turning from the battlements, he thought blackly that it was rather a pity that he didn't have a suicidal bone in his body.

Chapter 20

She tossed restlessly, hoping he would change his mind and seek her out to finish what they had begun. But she knew he wouldn't. Humankind made mating far too complicated. She wanted him, he wanted her. It should have been enough. *Damn him.*

Why couldn't he come to her on her terms, with passion and sweetness instead of rules and worries? But he wanted to lure her from a place of safety into a world that was too often merciless. Becoming "normal" would mean surrendering what had saved her.

And yet...in the heat of the moment, she had wanted to speak to him. Form her lips in unfamiliar ways to tell him how pleasing he was to her eyes, and how his presence delighted her. She wanted to ask more about his life, find what made him different from others. Perhaps, even, to tell him some of what had shaped her. Not the dark pieces that were best left in the shadows, but stories that would make his eyes laugh just for her.

Yet she could not speak, for doing so would change her life irrevocably.

Dominic awoke at dawn and found Meriel's ginger cat on his bed, watching him with eyes that glowed eerily in the faint light. If he believed in witches, he'd say the beast was her familiar, and had been sent to keep a watchful eye on him. Not believing in witches, he petted the cat, which promptly rolled onto its back so he could rub the soft belly. The creature was huge. Probably it had some wild cat in its ancestry. Maybe it was Meriel's *witchy familiar.*

Leaving the animal purring, he washed up and began to dress. During his fitful sleep, he'd developed a vague plan for resolving the situation with a minimum of damage. If Meriel voluntarily refused to wed Kyle, Amworth would not force her. Kyle would be upset, but as long as he didn't feel personally betrayed, he'd recover quickly. There was no shortage of other brides, almost any of which would suit him better than Meriel. God willing, Kyle would soon find himself another, more eligible female to marry. Once his affections were fixed elsewhere, Dominic could ask for Meriel's hand.

But the plan was riddled with weaknesses. When Dominic eventually courted Meriel, Kyle might feel betrayed anyhow. Or he might not seek another bride for years. Plus, Dominic would have to tell Amworth his real identity, and the longer he delayed, the harder it would be. Worst of all, he'd have to confess to Meriel, then enlist her cooperation in refusing Kyle and waiting for himself.

Would she do that? She was attracted to him, but that wasn't love. If what Meriel felt for him was merely the normal awakening of a young woman's desire, Kyle might do equally well. Gods above, Dominic would never be able to bear seeing them together! Emigrating to America would probably be necessary for his sanity.

As he finished dressing and left his room, he gloomily contemplated a range of possibilities, most ending dismally. All the more reason to work toward resolving the situation in a way that would benefit all concerned.

The first step was making peace with Meriel. Last night, she'd been ready to scratch his eyes out.

According to the groom, she had gone riding very early the last several mornings, before Warfield awoke. With luck, she would be riding again today.

Sure enough, when he reached the stables he found Meriel preparing to saddle Moonbeam. She saw him and stiffened, the saddle in her hands. He gave her a cheerful smile. "Good morning. May I ride with you?"

As he approached, he saw mixed emotions in her eyes. Pleasure at his arrival, combined with a strong desire to hurl the saddle at him. Holding her gaze, he said quietly, "I want there to be a future for us, Meriel, but it won't be easily won. I hope you're willing to work with me toward that."

Her eyes widened, and the stiffness went out of her posture. She didn't protest when he took the saddle from her hands and set it on Moonbeam, though her expression was puzzled. As he tightened the cinches, he said, "That split skirt is a good practical garment for riding. I assume one of the ladies made it. They take good care of you."

He cupped his hands to help her onto her mount, steeling himself not to be distracted by her nearness. When she stepped onto his linked hands, he found that she wore boots. He was glad of that; though she'd managed with bare feet, boots were definitely preferable.

She settled lightly on the mare's back, gathering the reins in one hand. With the other, she touched his cheek, rueful amusement in her eyes. He was forgiven.

Unable to entirely control himself, he caught her hand and kissed it swiftly. "I'll saddle Pegasus now. Wait for me?"

She smiled enigmatically and walked Moonbeam from the stables. Not sure if she would wait, he saddled his mount quickly and led the horse outside. He was pleased to find that she was walking the mare quietly around the courtyard.

As he swung into his own saddle, he said, "Do you have some special place you like to visit? If so, I'd be pleased to see it."

She set off at a fast trot. He followed, immensely relieved that they were on comfortable terms again. Later today, or perhaps tomorrow, he would explain who he really was and declare himself. She might turn out to be entirely indifferent to the fact that he wasn't Lord Maxwell.

Of course, it was equally possible she would be enraged to learn that he had been deceiving her. He'd simply have to take one fence at a time.

She led him up to the ancient standing stones that crowned a hill at the farthest, wildest corner of the park. Renbourne's reaction would tell her much about him.

On the way, he chatted with her easily. She liked that he spoke to her as an equal. Most people talked at her or over her, as if she were made of wood. She also enjoyed the way he could carry on both sides of a conversation quite nicely without her help.

But his gilded tongue fell silent when they neared their destination. Where they emerged from the woods, the stones stood stark and menacing against the early morning sky. She dismounted and tethered Moonbeam before entering the circle. Wordlessly Renbourne did the same.

He walked to the center of the circle and turned slowly, studying the irregularly shaped stones. Half a dozen had fallen, but three times as many still stood, looming to twice his height in silent testament to a race long vanished. He'd called her a pagan the night before, and she supposed he was right. Certainly she heard the old gods whisper when she came to this place.

He crossed to the tallest stone and laid his hands flat on the rough, lichened surface. After a long moment, he turned and said in a hushed voice, "This is a place of power, isn't it? Like a cathedral, one can feel the pulse of faith beating here."

He felt it, too! She wanted to kiss him for his perception, but refrained rather than risk offending his gentlemanly modesty.

"People must still come here," he said thoughtfully. "It can't be an accident that no trees grow inside the circle, or for several yards around outside."

She blinked. That had never occurred to her. Perhaps the circle was not as abandoned as she had thought. She liked the idea that some of the locals still held a place in their hearts for the old ways.

The rising sun was behind him, and his broad-shouldered silhouette made her think of a warrior, or perhaps a powerful priest. She shivered, touched by an uncanny feeling that the two of them had met here before. Perhaps her bones remembered lady ancestors who had brought their lovers here.

She bent and plucked a daisy from the grass by her feet. In the language of flowers, a symbol of innocence and gentleness. In the herbal written by a Meriel of three hundred years earlier, it was called Herb Margaret. The herbal had given the recipe for a salve made of daisies, good for wounds and bruises. Had that ancestress brought her sweetheart here and lain with him among the flowers?

Meriel tucked the daisy in one of his buttonholes, then flattened her hand in the middle of his chest, feeling the beat of his heart quicken under her touch. He covered her hand with his, saying huskily, "You belong in this place, my wild fairy maid."

She held her breath, hopeful that he might give in to the temptation visible in his eyes. The circle had an untamed pagan energy from the days long before the Christian god had commanded chastity. Who knew where a kiss might lead?

To her disappointment, he touched her hair so lightly she could scarcely feel it, then led the way back to the horses. She admired a man of firm resolve, but wished it were less firm in this case.

Nonetheless, the ride back to the house was pleasant. She had grown very accustomed to having him around.

The groom was awake, and he took charge of the horses when they reached the stables. Hungry from the exercise, she decided to join Renbourne in the breakfast parlor rather than beg tea and toast in the kitchen as she usually did.

He opened the door for her, and she swept by him. She'd noticed it was easier to sweep impressively when wearing boots. Renbourne murmured, "Well done, Lady Meriel! A princess could not have looked more regal."

She smiled, amused that he had interpreted her movements so accurately. Then she saw Mrs. Rector, and her smile faded. The older woman was perched on a bench in the hall, her face ashen as she read a letter that must have been delivered by the dusty messenger who stood awkwardly nearby.

Hearing their footsteps, Mrs. Rector looked up, her vision unfocused. Renbourne asked, "Is something wrong?"

"I'm afraid so." She ran her tongue over dry lips. "Lord Amworth has suffered a seizure of the heart. His wife, Elinor, says that...that the physician is not optimistic about the chances of his recovery." Her gaze dropped to the letter again. "He's my cousin, you know. I...I've known him my whole life."

A chill went through Meriel, and not only

because she, too, was fond of Lord Amworth. In her bones she knew this news would have repercussions that would shake her world.

The message about Lord Amworth cast a shadow over the household. Though earlier Dominic had hoped to work in the garden with Meriel, he was relieved when she vanished. He spent the day on the endless chore of trimming topiary chess pieces while he pondered the implications if Lord Amworth didn't recover.

Amworth himself had feared for Meriel if he died, because Lord Grahame's opinions on her best interests were so different from his own. A pity Dominic knew little about the law, and even less of the legal provisions surrounding Meriel's guardianship and inheritance. He simply did not know how much control her childhood guardians still had over her person. One thing was sure—Dominic had no standing on her behalf.

Upright and inflexible, Grahame would surely take a dim view of his niece's marriage to a younger son of small fortune. In fact, he would probably object to any marriage, and he'd be furious that Amworth had gone behind his back to arrange one.

Technically, Meriel was of age and free to make up her own mind, but Grahame might be able to get her declared incompetent if she chose to behave in a manner he considered mad. Though Dominic was sure that her mind and judgment were basically sound, as long as she didn't speak and behaved eccentrically, she was at risk of being treated as if she really were mad.

Would she speak up to preserve her freedom? Or would she withdraw into her own world and confirm the general belief that her wits were addled?

Uneasily Dominic recognized that a crisis was imminent. He must ask the ladies if they knew when Grahame was due back from his Continental journey. And he'd better pray that Amworth made a swift and unexpected recovery from his heart seizure.

When the members of the household gathered in the salon before dinner, Dominic was pleased to see that not only had Meriel appeared, but she was demurely dressed in one of her mother's gowns. She even wore soft kidskin slippers, slightly scuffed.

Both of the ladies smiled at the sight, which made him suspect that Meriel had made a special effort to cheer them up. Though Mrs. Marks was related to Meriel's father, not her mother, she had known Amworth for years and was almost as upset at his condition as Mrs. Rector was.

The butler poured sherry for each of them. Even Meriel took a glass, though Dominic had noticed that she drank virtually no alcohol.

Mrs. Rector moved to Dominic's side. "She looks so charming tonight. So...so normal. You've been very good for her, my lord."

"I hope so." He sipped his sherry. "But if

she looks elegant and ladylike, it's because she has been shown such fine examples through the years."

Mrs. Rector's eyes sparkled. "You've a silver tongue, my lord."

He was about to reply when a commotion sounded outside, in the front hall. A deep voice boomed, "Nonsense, of course they'll see me. D'you know who I am?"

The footman's reply was inaudible, but heavy approaching footsteps were heard, along with the visitor's comment, "Would've been here earlier if the cursed carriage hadn't broken an axle."

Dominic lowered his glass, his blood turning cold. No, it couldn't be. Surely it was just a similarity of voices....

The door to the salon swung open, and a broad man of implacable confidence swept into the room. Appalled, Dominic recognized the sixth Earl of Wrexham, and the slender, dark-haired young woman who trailed behind.

His father and sister had just arrived.

Chapter 21

Mrs. Marks stepped forward, her brows arched with polite challenge. "Good evening, sir. Do we have the pleasure of your acquaintance?"

Why the devil did everyone drop into Warfield unannounced? Thanking heaven for his father's notoriously bad eyesight, Dominic took a firm hold of Kyle's mannerisms, then drawled, "My apologies, Mrs. Marks, I didn't realize that you and my father were unacquainted. Mrs. Marks, Mrs. Rector, allow me to present the Earl of Wrexham and my sister, Lady Lucia Renbourne."

Adjusting swiftly, Mrs. Marks said, "What a pleasant surprise. Let me ring the housekeeper to prepare rooms for you." A delicate edge showed in her voice as she tugged the bellpull. "What a pity we couldn't have them ready."

Wrexham recognized her irritation but merely shrugged. "We were on our way north, and I decided I wanted to see how Maxwell was doing with his courting." His gaze swung to Meriel. "A pretty little thing. Doesn't look mad."

Meriel had drifted back to one wall, her gaze blank. Grateful for once that she didn't talk because he was afraid of what she might say, Dominic said hastily, "You must be tired from your journey. Would you like a glass of sherry?"

"I wouldn't say no to some brandy."

Dominic moved toward the drinks cabinet, hoping the ladies wouldn't mind that he was acting as host. "Lucia?"

"My usual." Lucia's apologetic gaze went to her hostesses with a sweet earnestness that could touch the hardest heart. "Mrs. Marks, Mrs. Rector, I'm so sorry that we've come at an awkward time."

Mrs. Marks's expression softened. "It's no

trouble, my dear. I'll simply have dinner set back an hour."

"No, no. We'll just finish our drinks, then take trays in our rooms." Wrexham covered a yawn. "No wish to put you out more than we already have. We'll stay through tomorrow and be off the next morning."

Dominic noted wryly that his father didn't consult Lucia about her dining preferences, or the ladies about whether they minded having uninvited guests for two nights. The charitable interpretation was that Wrexham thought of the families as already joined in marriage, but it was probably more accurate to say that it simply never occurred to him that anyone might object to his wishes.

As he poured the brandy, Dominic wondered what his sister's usual drink might be; she'd still been in the schoolroom when he'd left Dornleigh. Once she'd been fond of lemonade, but he didn't see any, nor any other beverage that he remembered her enjoying. Hoping for the best, he poured a sherry and crossed the room with the drinks.

Engaged in polite conversation with Mrs. Marks, his father accepted the brandy without looking up, but Lucia frowned when he gave her the other glass. "Sherry, Kyle?"

Then she raised her gaze. Slowly her eyes rounded, and the glass almost dropped from her hand. There was nothing wrong with Lucia's vision, and there wasn't a prayer that Dominic could fool her. She'd have recognized

236

him immediately if she hadn't been expecting to see Kyle.

Turning his back so that she was the only one in the room who could see, he touched his finger to his lips, his eyes pleading for her cooperation. She swallowed and took a firmer grip on the stem of her glass, her gaze darting to her father.

Voice almost inaudible, Dominic murmured, "A good thing he's too vain to wear his spectacles. There's a sound reason for this, I swear."

Lucia regarded her brother sternly. "There had better be."

"I'll explain later," he promised. Then he slid away, grateful that she hadn't given him away. Yet.

Dominic was relieved when his father and sister withdrew to their newly prepared rooms, but he could still feel his father's presence in the house like a thundercloud. Though he was safe for this evening, what about tomorrow? Wrexham's vision might be weak, but he wasn't stupid. If Dominic couldn't discuss topics familiar to Kyle and the earl, he'd be caught, and there would be holy hell to pay.

It was hard to enjoy dinner when his mind persisted in counting the number of people who would be outraged to learn the truth. In fact, Dominic couldn't think of anyone who *wouldn't* be shocked.

Meriel disappeared after the meal, and Dominic excused himself from the drawing room early. It was a kindness, really, because with him gone the ladies could discuss the Renbourne invasion freely.

The footman on duty directed him upstairs to his sister's room. There he tapped on the door, half hoping she'd be asleep, but she called out, "Come in."

He opened the door and stepped inside. Clad in a flowing blue robe, Lucia sat on a stool in front of the dressing table while her maid brushed her hair. Turning, she gave her brother a baleful glance. "Jane, you may go now."

She waited for the door to close behind her maid before asking, "What on earth is going on, Dominic?"

He crossed the room to her. "I'll explain, but don't you have a hug for your prodigal brother first?"

"Of course." Her expression relaxed into a smile as she rose and embraced him. "It's been too long since you came home, Dom. But what a wicked prank this is! I've spent the evening worrying about how much trouble you'll be in if you're discovered." She pulled away, a furrow between her brows. "You do have a good reason, don't you?"

"Why am I not surprised that I'm the one being blamed for this?" Dominic said wryly as he sat on the canopied bed. "It's simple, really. Kyle had some other pressing engagement—he wouldn't say what—so he asked me to come in his place."

"Kyle asked you to help him, and you agreed," Lucia repeated incredulously as she dropped onto the stool again. "And you say that's simple? You've hardly spoken to each other in years."

"Which is why it's obvious that this is very important to him." Dominic hesitated a moment, wondering how much to say. Deciding that if he was going to ask his sister to lie for him, she deserved the truth, he continued, "I don't know what he's doing, but I believe he's left the country. He only intended to be gone for a few weeks, though."

Lucia started twisting her long hair into a rope. "Why did you agree? Did you think it would be amusing to deceive two sweet old ladies and a girl who is deranged?"

"Lucia!" He propelled himself from the bed and began pacing the room, thinking that his sister was becoming entirely too cynical. But of course, she had been moving in London society for several years. That tended to take the edge off innocence very quickly. "Believe me, I'm no happier about this deception than you are. I did it for two reasons. First, Kyle has offered to give me Bradshaw Manor if I manage to impersonate him successfully."

Lucia's eyes widened. "Heavens, he really *was* serious. I can see why that would be a hard offer to refuse." She cocked her head. "And the other reason?"

He hesitated, wishing he had restricted himself to real estate. "Because he seemed so...so desperate. As if he'd break from the pressure if I didn't agree to help."

"He has seemed upset lately," she agreed. "I've been worried, but of course he wouldn't tell his little sister what was wrong even if I'd dared to ask."

"Kyle could give a rock lessons in silence." He'd kept things from Dominic, too, creating another wedge between them after they were sent to separate schools. During the holidays, Dominic talked about his lessons and new friends, trying to maintain the fabric of their relationship. But Kyle hadn't been interested in Dominic's life.

Lucia regarded Dominic gravely. "I'm glad you care about him enough to help. I've never understood why you two are so estranged. It seems as if twins ought to like each other. You did once."

He stopped pacing and stared out the window. The room faced the front lawn, where moonlight illuminated the sweeping drive. "I've never disliked Kyle. I'm not sure the reverse is true."

"Oh, he cares about you," Lucia said softly. "And resents that you've turned your back on him. Just as you resent the fact that he's the heir and you're not."

He spun on his heel and glared at his sister. She had definitely grown up. He thought longingly of when she had been ten, with grass stains on her skirt and her hair every which way. She'd loved her big brothers quite uncritically then. "I didn't ask for your opinion on my relationship with Kyle."

She smiled sweetly. "I know. That's why I thought I'd better volunteer it."

"Mistress Mischief rides again," he said, resurrecting her childhood nickname. "Enough about me. Have you any exciting news?"

She blushed, her worldly air falling away. "I'm betrothed."

"Really!" he said, delighted. "I missed seeing the notices in the newspapers."

"The formal announcement hasn't been made yet." She shook her twisted hair free. "Actually, that's why Papa and I are here. We're on our way to Robert's family in Lancashire. The notices will be sent after the settlements are signed."

Dominic grinned. "And you'd rather be there instead of wasting time in Shropshire. Wrexham must be glad you finally accepted someone. Another year or two, and you'd be on the shelf."

She laughed. "You're right, Papa is much relieved, even though he's not enthusiastic about the match. He keeps muttering that I could have done better than the son of a mere baron."

"Obviously you don't think so." He picked up one of the small glass cosmetic jars from his sister's dressing table. Did Meriel have pretty little feminine trinkets like these? Would she want them? "Who's the lucky man? Some handsome devil, I'm sure."

Lucia leaned forward on her stool eagerly. "Robert Justice, Lord Justice's heir. He isn't exactly handsome, not like you and Kyle, but Robin has such a twinkle in his eyes, and he's so wonderful to talk to, and..." She broke off, blushing again.

"And wonderful to kiss, I daresay." Dominic searched his memory, and a solid, brown-haired young man with an easy smile came to mind. Not showy, but good for the long haul. Lucia had sound judgment. He hugged her again. "I wish you happy, little sister. I've met him once or twice. He's a good fellow."

"I know." Lucia's voice was muffled against his shoulder. Emerging from his embrace, she continued, "What about Lady Meriel? Do you think she'll make Kyle happy? There are some very...very odd stories about her."

He stiffened at the reminder that Meriel was destined for Kyle. "She's unusual, but very...charming. If Kyle takes the time to really get to know her, I'm sure they'll deal well together."

Lucia nodded, clearly unconvinced. "She's rather pretty, though her gown was terribly out of date."

Dominic bit back a desire to point out that Meriel was not merely pretty but beautiful, and that a gown that had been handsome twenty years earlier was handsome still. If he said that, his too-perceptive sister might notice that his feelings were not exactly brotherly. "She has no need of a new wardrobe in the country, but she has skills other than fashion. For example, she's a wonderful gardener. Also, in India she learned how to paint interesting henna decorations on the skin." He grinned. "Perhaps you should ask her to draw Robert's name in a place where not just anyone would see it."

"Dominic, you have a low mind." Lucia's eyes narrowed pensively. "Still...the designs are temporary?"

"Yes. I promise you that Robert would be most intrigued." He covered a yawn. "Time I went to bed. I need my rest if I'm to persuade Wrexham that I'm really Kyle tomorrow. I was never very good at dealing with him."

"Papa really isn't so bad, Dom, except when his gout is hurting him," she said earnestly. "Just be more patient. If you lose your temper and stamp off, you'll give yourself away. Kyle is always very cool and polite, even when Papa is being difficult."

Dominic had always had more freedom to lose his temper and leave when Wrexham was being impossible. As the heir, Kyle had been forced to stay and endure. For the first time, it occurred to Dominic to wonder if his brother came by his rigid control naturally, or if it had evolved out of the necessity of dealing with the earl. "Will you keep silent, Lucia? I know it's a lot to ask, but if Wrexham realizes what we've done...." Dominic made an expressive gesture.

"I won't tell. I don't want to even think about the unpleasantness that would result if Papa discovers you aren't Kyle." She caught her breath. "The valets! Papa's Wilcox must have already seen your valet in the servants' hall."

"Kyle lent me Morrison. He doesn't want Kyle to get into trouble, either."

"Then you might be able to carry this off. Try to say as little as possible." Lucia shook her head. "But what about later? Surely the next time Kyle comes to Warfield, people will notice the difference."

Dominic shrugged. "I said the same thing, but he wasn't concerned. He thought that the opinions of Mrs. Rector and Mrs. Marks and the servants didn't matter, and Lady Meriel wouldn't know the difference."

Lucia sniffed. "Do you believe that?"

"I have to hope he's right." Uneasily Dominic considered the future. Exchanging twins would probably work if months passed between Dominic's departure and Kyle's appearance. But if the marriage were to take place before Lord Grahame returned, there wouldn't be enough time for memories to become obscured.

Damnation, he didn't *want* Kyle to marry Meriel. Yet if Dominic revealed their deception now, the situation would only get worse.

Mind chasing in futile circles, he bid his sister good night and went to bed.

Meriel waited until a few minutes after Renbourne had left his sister's room. Then she took a flower arrangement to the bedroom door and knocked. Seeing Jena Ames again had sharpened her curiosity about other young women. Especially one who was Renbourne's sister.

Lady Lucia opened the door. She shared her brother's dark brown hair and blue eyes. Though she was inches taller than Meriel and very grand, the two girls were probably about the same age. "Oh! Good evening, Lady Meriel."

Meriel held out her floral offering, a tall glass cylinder once used for storage in the pantry. Now it held clusters of fragrant lilac and trailing vines of dark, glossy ivy. Meriel had deliberately made the bouquet rather conventional, since she doubted that a London lady would appreciate one of her wilder creations. Renbourne was the only one who'd ever really understood her arrangements.

Lucia took the vase with a pleased smile. "Why, thank you." She buried her pretty nose in lilac blossoms. "How lovely this smells." Glancing up, she said, "Would you like to come in? Since we are going to be sisters-in-law, I should like to become better acquainted." She stepped back and made a welcoming gesture.

Meriel had hoped for such an invitation. With someone else she might have simply entered the room without being asked, but she didn't want Renbourne's sister to dislike her. Odd to care what a stranger thought; she wasn't sure she liked the experience, but there it was. She did care.

Lucia set the flowers on her bedside table, then turned, expression uncertain. "I'm told you can't speak, and I...I don't know quite how to behave. Please excuse me if I accidentally offend you. I don't mean to."

Meriel liked her for her directness. Truly Renbourne's sister. She made a small gesture encouraging Lucia to talk.

The other woman dropped onto the bed in a swirl of blue silk. "It's not official yet, but I'm to be married soon. Papa and I are on our way to visit my betrothed and his family in Lancashire." She looked hopeful. "May I tell you about him? My father thinks I'm silly to want to talk about Robin all the time, but another female might understand."

Meriel had to smile. Donning an expression of interest, she settled into the sofa as Lady Lucia began to describe the manifold wonders of the Honorable Robert Justice. The glow on her face was intriguing. A sign of being in love, apparently.

Did Lucia also feel the fierce physical craving that drew Meriel to Renbourne? If so, she was too well bred to show it. But passion might well be the fuel behind the tumbling words and sparkling eyes.

Eventually Lucia stopped and gave a deprecatory laugh. "Sorry, I'm talking your ears off. You're very patient to indulge me." Absently she leaned against the carved bedpost. "I hope you come to love my brother as I love Robin. I think of him all the time. Though we'll be married in early autumn, I can scarcely endure the waiting."

Meriel looked away, not wishing to show the other girl what lived in her own eyes. She did not understand love or marriage, and she was having precious little luck learning about passion. But she knew what it was to think of a man constantly.

Lucia interrupted her thoughts, her voice hesitant. "My brother said that you know how to paint henna designs on the skin. I thought it sounded...very interesting." Her voice rose questioningly at the end.

Meriel stood and crossed the room, rolling back her right sleeve as she did. On her wrist was a delicately traced bracelet of linked paisley patterns.

"How charming." Lucia carefully touched the henna design, as if fearing she would damage it. "My brother says this is temporary?"

Meriel nodded, thinking that they were having a true conversation even though she responded with gestures, not words. It seemed safe because Lucia would be leaving soon and not give her away. She had to admit that Renbourne was right—a conversation was more enjoyable when both parties participated, but she wasn't sure she was ready to let her usual circle of people know how much she understood.

The other girl blushed. "Would you be willing...would you mind...putting a design on my shoulder? Where it would be covered by a gown." She indicated the area she meant. "And if you did...could it include the initials R and L?"

Meriel almost laughed aloud. So the grand young lady wanted to surprise her intended. Passion was definitely part of Lucia's love. Had Renbourne suggested that a man would be intrigued by a hidden design? If so, did that mean he would be?

Meriel gestured to Lucia to wait, then returned to her room to mix a bowl of henna. She liked Renbourne's sister.

And Lucia had given her a most interesting idea....

Chapter 22

Kind sea winds brought them swiftly to Cádiz, a city of white turrets that rose from the sea like a shining dream. Though Constancia had been raised in the north of Spain, far from the coast, she had visited Cádiz and never forgotten the city's beauty.

Kyle paced along the seafront promenade, wishing she were beside him, but she was resting under the balm of laudanum.

Too restless to spend all day in the villa, *waiting,* he had chosen to explore the city on foot. The lofty buildings and squares were haunted by the ghostly presence of the Phoenician traders who had founded Cádiz three thousand years earlier, and the Romans who had made the city a great imperial port. More recently, Cádiz had been the Spanish colonial gateway, with the wealth of the Americas pouring into its coffers.

Best of all were the promenades that fringed the great Atlantic harbor. As he watched the ships sail in and out, his excitement was underlaid by corrosive guilt at finding such pleasure in the city when Constancia lay dying. Yet he could not still the race of his blood at hearing sailors shouting in a dozen strange tongues, nor could he suppress his speculation about what distant lands these ships had seen.

The scents of the port still tingled in his nostrils as he returned to the villa. It was a handsome place, owned by a London friend who had grown rich shipping sherry from Cádiz. Wrexham didn't approve of having merchants for friends, but Kyle found that such men were usually more interesting than the nobles of his own class.

He had just entered the cool tiled hall of the villa when Constancia's maid, Teresa, raced up to him. "My lord!" she gasped, her eyes huge and dark. "Come quickly!"

Oh, God, no, not yet. Not so soon. Heart hammering, he raced past the maid to Constancia's room, which opened onto the courtyard garden. The scent of orange blossoms wafted through the windows, painfully alive in contrast to Constancia's utter stillness. For a horrible moment he feared she was dead, until she drew a slow, harshly rattling breath.

He took her hand, as if he could call her back from whatever distant place she had gone. "Teresa, has the physician been called?"

"Sí, my lord. But I do not know when he will come."

Unable to just watch helplessly, he ordered, "Bring brandy and a spoon."

Grateful to have passed responsibility to him, Teresa obeyed. Then, while Kyle prayed that spirits would stimulate Constancia, the maid carefully spooned brandy between her mistress's lips, a few drops at a time so she wouldn't choke.

Constancia's lids fluttered up, revealing dark exhausted eyes. "I have worried you, querido," she murmured. "Forgive me."

He exhaled a sigh of relief. "No matter, as long as you are still here."

She squeezed his hand with a pressure so light he could barely feel it. "My time...has not yet come. I will tell you when to send for the priest."

He smiled at her, but inside he was still quaking. Instinctively he sensed that she had been very, very near to passing away. And he wasn't ready to let her go yet.

He wasn't ready.

Chapter 23

Vaguely hoping he could disappear into the gardens and avoid his father for most of the day, Dominic rose early, but he didn't have the breakfast parlor to himself for long. He'd barely surveyed the dishes on the sideboard before other members of the household began to appear.

First came Mrs. Marks, followed shortly by Mrs. Rector. Then Meriel, looking so well behaved that he wondered what she was up to.

She cast a demure sideways glance as she served herself coddled eggs and toast, then sat opposite him at the table. Her manners were impeccable when she chose to exercise them.

Lucia appeared, eyes sparkling. As she passed Dominic, she said under her breath, "Lady Meriel's henna designs are wonderful!" Then she moved on, gaily greeting the ladies and Meriel before he could learn more.

The group was actually quite convivial, until the Earl of Wrexham appeared. A pall of silence fell over the breakfast parlor. Dominic silently cursed himself for not eating more quickly.

His father was limping, a sign that his gout was acting up, but he said with gruff good cheer, "Morning. Nothing like a sound night's sleep after a long journey." He glanced out the window. "A pleasant day. Good for viewing the estate."

Dominic was tempted to point out that it was vulgar to let his lust for Meriel's acres show so much, but he held his tongue, as Kyle would have.

"Good morning, Lord Wrexham." Mrs. Marks started to rise.

The earl waved her back. "Don't interrupt your meal on my behalf. I'll just help myself." After collecting a substantial mound of eggs, ham, deviled kidneys, sliced tongue, and toast, he limped to the table. Meriel ignored him, but Dominic saw her draw inward when the earl set his plate next to her.

Instead of sitting himself, Wrexham studied

Meriel's downcast profile. "She's a pretty puss. A pity she's so small, but she seems healthy enough. Come, look at me."

He grasped her chin and raised her face. Her eyes flashed and she jerked her head away, not letting their gazes connect. Wrexham laughed. "Here, girl, don't be shy. I want to see what my grandchildren will look like." He reached for her chin again.

Meriel bit his finger. Hard. A collective gasp rose around the table as everyone stared in shock.

"Bloody hell!" The earl snatched his hand back, his stunned expression turning to fury. "How dare you! Has no one ever taught you manners?"

Seeing his father's hand tighten into a fist, Dominic leaped from his chair and unobtrusively caught the older man's wrist. Keeping his voice smooth, as Kyle would, he said, "You startled her, sir."

He gave Meriel a swift glance. Eyes glittering, she looked ready to bite again. Dominic shifted his weight, moving his father a step farther away.

The interruption gave the earl time to regain his temper, but he glowered as he said, "Amworth assured me that the chit wasn't violent."

Irritated on Meriel's behalf, Dominic retorted, "Would you enjoy being handled like this by a stranger?" He grasped his father's chin, forcing the older man to look up into his eyes. It was startling to realize he was a full three inches taller. The earl always seemed larger, dominating any group he was in.

"Damn you, boy, you're worse than she is!" his father roared as he broke his son's grip. "How dare you raise a hand to me!"

Help arrived from an unexpected quarter when Lucia said brightly, "As Maxwell just demonstrated, it's not very pleasant to be treated like a horse whose teeth must be checked for wear, Papa." She gave her father a dazzling smile. "Though I know it's kindly meant, I can't tell you how often I've wished to bite aging dowagers and elderly gentlemen who pinched my cheeks and told me what a sweet creature I am." Glancing at Meriel, she said tolerantly, "Never having gone out in society, Lady Meriel hasn't learned that one really mustn't bite, no matter how tempted."

Rising from her chair, Lucia deftly transferred her father's plate to the empty place setting next to her own. "Here, Papa, come sit by me. The view of the gardens from this window is quite extraordinary." Taking his arm, she escorted him to the chair. "I'll get your coffee for you."

While Lucia performed her doting daughter role, Meriel turned and stalked from the breakfast parlor like an angry cat. Dominic could only be grateful that she and his father were no longer in the same room. But God help them all, the day had just begun.

Lucia's advice was sound; speaking only when it was unavoidable simplified Dominic's time with his father. They left the park and rode over the estate under the guidance of the steward. Kerr did most of the talking. Wrexham eyed the fields and grazing herds shrewdly, making occasional comments. Dominic was impressed. Having received most of his own agricultural instruction from the Dornleigh steward, he hadn't fully appreciated the depth of his father's knowledge.

After the tour they returned to the house in time to join the ladies for a light midday meal. Dominic concentrated on his plate rather than the conversation. When he finished, he considered slipping away, but doing so would be suspiciously discourteous, so he suggested to his father, "Would you like to walk in the gardens? They are Lady Meriel's particular interest, and quite splendid."

The earl hesitated, then shook his head. "I'll spend a quiet afternoon inside, away from the heat. You find that little hellcat you're courting, and teach her some manners."

Dominic's stab of irritation at the description of Meriel vanished when he looked at his father and saw him as if for the first time. Wrexham had married late and his sons had not been born right away, so he was nearing seventy. In the years since Dominic had left home to go into the army, the earl had gone from the prime of life to old age. A hazing of his eyes hinted at developing cataracts, and surely diminished hearing was part of the reason for his booming voice.

He'd gained considerable weight, too, and could no longer be considered merely stocky;

the Renbourne children had inherited their lean builds and athleticism from their mother. With the earl's age and weight, this morning's riding must have been very tiring. Yet just as he'd never spared his children, he'd never spared himself. He'd always taken his responsibilities as a landowner and a member of the House of Lords seriously, and had never indulged in the extravagance and debauchery common among men of his class.

Now fatigue and pain showed in the deep lines of his face. Though he had never been an easy man, he was worthy of respect. Is this how Kyle saw the earl, and the reason why he could be so patient?

Shaken by this insight, Dominic answered, "I shall tell Meriel that she is not to bite anyone again." Then he departed before his face could color at the vivid thoughts Meriel's name aroused in him.

As he was leaving the house, his sister caught up with him. "Will you show me around the gardens?" Though she didn't use his real name, there was hidden meaning in her voice when she added, "It seems like forever since I've seen you."

With a pang, he recognized how much he'd missed Lucia. He'd gone to her coming-out ball, of course, but their meetings since were chance encounters because he hadn't wished to call at Wrexham House and risk running into his father and brother. He offered his arm. "It would be my pleasure to show you the gardens."

As he guided her through the parterre, he

said quietly, "I'm sorry I haven't seen more of you, Lucia. I forgot how quickly little sisters grow up."

She shrugged philosophically. "I understood why you weren't comfortable at Dornleigh. It would have been like three stallions pawing and snorting under the same roof. It's bad enough just with Kyle and Papa sometimes. But I've missed you."

He picked a small blue flower and tucked it behind her ear. "By leaving the field to Kyle, I've assured that he has become your favorite brother," he said wryly.

She halted and scowled at him. "Stop that! Why do you think there's a competition? You're twins, but you're not the same. I know Kyle better because we've lived under the same roof most of our lives, but I love both of you equally."

He was taken aback, never having been snapped at by his sister. He thought about what she was saying. "I'm sorry, Lucia. Even at the best of times, Kyle and I were always competing, with neither of us really winning. Our abilities were too similar. It might have been easier if one of us was clearly superior. Instead, we were always jostling for position. But it's not fair of me to involve you in our private war, even as a joke."

"No, it isn't," she said tartly. "I want you both at my wedding, and acting like gentlemen."

"I'll be there, and I promise to behave." Although when he considered the explosive

256

possibilities inherent in his feelings for Meriel, he knew that Kyle might not feel so amiable. His stomach twisted. Lord, would Meriel and Kyle be married by then?

Stopping himself before his thoughts could start circling again, he turned onto a path that led to Meriel's tree house. Lucia gasped at the sight of the improbable structure perched in its oak tree. "How wonderful! Every child's dream. Have you been up in it?"

"It's Meriel's private sanctuary, and I've never been invited." As he scanned the tree, he had a mental image of Meriel playing the role of besieged castle owner and pouring boiling oil from the windows. He smiled at the thought. "Since the ladder isn't down, she's probably there now."

He took Lucia under the tree house in the hopes that Meriel might appear. His sister peered upward, shading her eyes against the sun. "I see there's a lock on the trapdoor. She's serious about privacy, isn't she?" Raising her voice, she called, "Meriel, are you there? Will you let us visit your tree house or join us for a walk?"

No answer. Dominic wasn't surprised. "She's probably still angry about what happened at breakfast." He took Lucia's arm and guided her across the clearing where he had lured Meriel from her tree to picnic.

"I don't blame her. As I said this morning, I've often wished to bite someone myself." Lucia grinned. "I'm glad she didn't really hurt Papa, but I do envy her the freedom to bite.

There is something to be said for being thought a little daft."

A little daft. He liked the sound of that much better than "mad." "You mentioned her henna painting. Did she show you the one on her wrist?"

Lucia nodded. "She brought me some flowers right after you left last night. We had a very nice visit. I told her all about Robin, and she drew a design on me."

Since this was his little sister, he decided that he didn't want to know where it had been placed. "I'll show you the topiary now. Warfield has the finest I've ever seen."

As he and Lucia strolled down the paths, he realized that the worst of his father's visit was over, and he hadn't been recognized yet. All he had to do was get through the evening. Since Meriel obviously didn't like the earl, she would probably skip dinner, which would reduce the opportunities for trouble. He was safe.

Yet for a treacherous moment, he considered what might happen if his father recognized that the wrong twin was courting Meriel. Might that be enough to cause Wrexham to withdraw his support for the betrothal? Hard to say; certainly he was impressed with the estate and dearly wanted to bring it into the family. One thing was sure: exposing the deception would cause havoc, and a public scandal if word got beyond the families involved.

His churning thoughts slowly crystallized into an unwelcome realization. He could no longer remain at Warfield, wanting Meriel more every day. Amworth and Wrexham had both visited and given their tacit blessings to the courtship, and Meriel had become accustomed to his presence. He'd done what Kyle wanted.

Now it was time to leave. Distance and diversion might diminish the spell Meriel had cast over him. Of course he was entranced by her—she was lovely, and the most intriguing creature he'd ever met. That didn't mean he was deeply in love with her. Separation would help him understand his feelings better.

He hated the thought so much that he knew it was the right decision.

Chapter 24

Dominic dressed for dinner with extra care, since it was to be more formal than usual in honor of the distinguished guests. He'd managed to escape detection so far. Just a few more hours, and he should be safe. He glanced over his shoulder at Morrison, who was collecting Dominic's razor and other toiletry articles. "You've seen my father's servants belowstairs. Have any suspicions been raised?"

Morrison shook his head. "None at all. You've done well, sir."

A compliment from Morrison! Amazing. If Dominic wasn't careful, his self-opinion would become quite overexalted.

As he headed downstairs to the salon, he planned his departure. Not tomorrow—it might seem odd if he left immediately after Wrexham and Lucia. But the next day, or the one after. Certainly by the end of the week.

Hell.

He was the last to reach the salon. After an afternoon of rest, his father was in good spirits, and all the ladies were looking their best. Lucia really was a remarkably fine-looking girl. And, blessedly, no Meriel. He regretted seeing so little of her today, but it was better that she didn't appear again until Wrexham was gone.

But then, Dominic would soon be gone, too. *Hell.*

Donning a smile, he accepted a glass of sherry and joined in the casual talk until the dinner bell rang. Mrs. Marks said, "Shall we go in to dine? Cook has made special efforts tonight."

Unhurriedly the guests prepared to move into the dining room. Then Meriel appeared in the hall doorway.

Dominic happened to be looking in that direction, so he was the first to notice her. He almost choked on his sherry. Lord, but the girl knew how to make an entrance!

Seeing his reaction, the others turned until all five sets of eyes were locked on Meriel. She was in costume again, her slim form swathed enticingly in translucent silk that shimmered between moonstone white and a pale green that emphasized the color of her eyes. One shoulder was bared, revealing an intricate henna medallion, while her silks were secured on the other shoulder by a grand, barbaric gold ornament. A pair of gold combs swept her hair above her ears before releasing it to cascade down her back.

When she had everyone's attention, she moved forward gracefully, her elegant bare feet visible below the swirl of silk. In fact, Dominic saw with fascination, the fabric was draped to include a slit on the right side so that each step allowed brief glimpses of calf and knee. A henna pattern ran upward from her ankle chain until it disappeared under the sari, causing irresistible speculations about how high it went.

Behind her walked the ginger cat, and then Roxana, the animals following with the dignity of royal retainers. How the devil did she manage to get a cat to do that?

"That's indecent!" Wrexham sputtered when he'd recovered from his shock. "Has the girl *no* sense of propriety?"

"She's wearing an Indian sari," Mrs. Rector explained imperturbably. "Quite unexceptional for a Hindu lady. Her mother collected foreign garments and jewelry, and Meriel enjoys wearing them on special occasions."

Dominic suspected that Meriel's version of a sari was more suitable to a dancing girl than a respectable lady, but it was very fetching indeed. The cluster of bangles on one slim wrist and the golden ankle chain visible when she walked added to her allure. To his father, he said, "Lady Meriel apparently wished to honor your visit, sir."

"You look splendid, Meriel," Lucia said warmly. "I wish I could wear such a garment, but I'm too tall and would look like a great gawk, I fear." Nonetheless, there was a gleam in her eyes that made Dominic wonder if Robert Justice might someday receive an exotic treat from his bride.

Looking suspiciously demure, Meriel bowed before each guest, her hands pressed together in front of her chest. Darkened lashes and brows increased the drama of her appearance. Dominic heard a faint chiming when she dipped in front of him, and saw that she'd replaced her usual silver moon earrings with dangling clusters of tiny gold bells.

Though her eyes were downcast, her movement revealed more glimpses of leg, and a tantalizing hint of rounded breasts. Dominic tried not to stare, but doubted that he was successful. She was luminous, a true fairy queen.

Wrexham scowled when she bowed before him. "No proper English lady comes to dinner wearing only an indecent pagan scarf."

"Surely in the privacy of her own home, she can wear the garments bequeathed by her mother," Dominic said blandly.

"Fit only for the bedroom," the earl muttered. Scowling, he offered Mrs. Marks his arm to lead her into the dining room.

Since the occasion was formal, Dominic took Mrs. Rector in to the dinner table, while the two young ladies followed, Lucia chatting happily to Meriel. She seemed to have accepted the idea of a mute sister-in-law very easily.

Dominic glanced over his shoulder and saw that the cat and dog completed the procession. He was half-surprised not to see Meriel's hedgehog bringing up the rear.

Suppressing a smile, he took Mrs. Rector to her chair. She and Mrs. Marks, as cohostesses, were seated at the ends of the table, with Wrexham and Meriel on one side and Lucia and Dominic opposite. The floral centerpiece was so conventional that it must have been done by one of the ladies.

He took his chair across from Meriel, glad that she seemed at ease even though the earl was beside her. Roxana flopped on the floor behind Meriel's chair, while the cat found a spot between Meriel and Mrs. Rector.

The serving of food and drink occupied the next few minutes. Dominic kept a wary eye on Meriel, hoping she'd behave herself until the meal was over. At least the earl knew better than to pinch her chin again.

The ladies and Lucia carried the conversation, with his sister recounting good-natured stories about the London Season. Otherwise it would have been a silent meal, since Dominic had resolved to say as little as possible and the earl was still scowling.

When Dominic first felt a touch on his foot, he thought the cat was wandering. Then the pressure became a gentle caress up the inside of his ankle. After a startled moment, he realized that Meriel was stroking him with her bare foot.

He stared, amazed, but her attention was on her plate. Not so much as a flicker of an eyelash indicated that the little minx was misbehaving. He drew his feet back and crossed them under his chair, out of reach.

For a while she left him in peace. Then, as the first course was removed and the plates and china changed in preparation for the second course, he once again felt a soft pressure, this time on the inside of his knee. He stiffened, unable to suppress the surge of desire that blazed through him. Meriel had the uninhibited sensuality of a first-class courtesan. Either that, or a diabolical sense of humor. Probably both.

He'd almost collected himself again when a light pinch on his thigh almost sent him jumping out of his skin. How the devil had Meriel reached so far? Then he realized that Lucia had pinched him in an attempt to get his attention.

When he turned to his sister, she gave him a warning glance. "Yes, do tell us your plans for the wedding."

He swallowed hard, wondering who had asked the original question that Lucia was repeating for his benefit. "To be honest, I haven't thought much on the subject. Meriel's uncle Amworth is ill, you know. Since he is her guardian, it would be inappropriate to make plans for the time being."

Mrs. Rector looked up from her lamb collops. "I forgot to tell you that I received a letter from Lady Amworth today. Apparently

Amworth has rallied a bit. His condition is still grave, but..." She sighed. "It is impossible not to hope."

"That's good news." Dominic uttered a fervent mental prayer that Amworth would recover. Certainly the man's survival would improve his niece's situation.

As the conversation turned to Amworth's sons, whom Lucia knew from London, Meriel's foot slid between Dominic's thighs and nestled warmly over his genitals. He gasped, and hardened instantly. God in heaven, he'd never get through this dinner! He wanted desperately to sweep the little witch into his arms and carry her off to the nearest bedroom and make frantic love to her.

After a few crazed moments of lustful thoughts, he managed to reestablish a semblance of control. A good thing Lucia was in such fine form tonight. Her stories were keeping the ladies laughing and covering up his own distraction. He guessed that she was making a special effort to keep attention away from him.

He glanced at his father, which had a sobering effect, before looking at Meriel. She'd had to sink down in her seat to extend her foot under the full breadth of the table. He unobtrusively moved his chair back a few inches. That helped, but her wicked little toes could still reach his inner thighs. He reached under the table and caught her foot with one hand. A wonderful foot, strong and well-shaped and remarkably deft.

Meriel raised her gaze from her plate and

regarded him with slumberous eyes. The girl was downright dangerous. Hoping rather desperately that she was ticklish, he drew his fingernail lightly along the arch of her foot. She made a sound reminiscent of a mouse squeak and jerked her foot away. He took the opportunity to move his chair back again, taking himself completely out of Meriel's range.

When she scowled at him, he grinned. A spark of answering humor showed in her eyes before she dropped her gaze again. She knew perfectly well how outrageously she was behaving, and was enjoying every minute of his discomfiture.

Wrexham, who had spoken little while steadily emptying his wineglass, said abruptly, "The sooner you marry the girl and take control of the property, Maxwell, the better. The steward seems a competent fellow, but unimaginative. With better management, you can realize at least five hundred pounds a year more in income."

Since his gaze was on Meriel, Dominic saw her go rigid at his father's words. Guessing that she didn't like the idea of her property being so casually claimed, he said, "It's premature to discuss changes at Warfield when the marriage is not yet fully confirmed." He regarded Meriel with foreboding. "Lady Meriel must be willing— Amworth insists on that, and I agree."

"She looks willing to me." The earl raked Meriel with a fulminating glance. "The sooner she's wedded and bedded and got with child, the better."

As Meriel's pale skin turned scarlet, Dominic said tightly, "You forget yourself, sir. Such talk is not fitting in this company."

"Nonsense." Wrexham tilted his wineglass toward his hostesses in an informal salute. "Mrs. Marks and Mrs. Rector are widows, and both of the girls are on the verge of marriage." He frowned at Meriel. "And not a minute too soon. Amworth should have married the chit off years ago. I don't envy you the job of controlling her. You'll have to keep her on a tight rein to ensure that the heir to Wrexham is of Renbourne blood."

As Mrs. Marks uttered a protest, Meriel rose from her chair and glared at the earl. Holding his gaze, she lifted her claret-filled wineglass by the stem, then whipped it downward to smash on the edge of the table. The sound of shattering crystal filled the air as blood-crimson wine sprayed across the white linen tablecloth.

Her head swung around toward Dominic, and he saw hurt as well as rage in her eyes. Then she bolted from the dining room, her silken sari flaring behind her.

"What the devil got into her?" the earl sputtered.

Dominic leaped to his feet. So furious he could barely speak, he spat out, "Congratulations, Lord Wrexham. You've managed with a few insults to destroy all of my efforts to build a relationship with Lady Meriel. If you truly want this marriage, you've picked a damnable way of showing it." He rounded the table to go after Meriel...

And almost broke his neck tripping over Roxana, who planted herself in front of him just before he reached the door. Swearing, he managed to catch the door frame and save himself from crashing ignominiously to the floor.

He glared down at the dog, who regarded him with a curled lip and apologetic eyes. The poor brute wanted to protect her mistress, but she liked Dominic.

Ignoring his father, Dominic knelt by Roxana and held out his hand, forcing his thoughts into calmer channels. After several uncertain moments, the dog licked his palm, friends once more. He gave her a quick head scratch, then went out the door, closing it quickly so that Roxana couldn't follow.

Naturally Meriel had vanished from the corridor by this time. He tried to think where she might have gone. The house was large enough to provide dozens of hiding places, but he doubted she was here. Her instincts usually sent her outdoors, into the sanctuary of Warfield Park, where she could probably hide forever if she chose.

Sanctuary. Guessing that the tree house was her most likely retreat, he swiftly left the house and headed for the great oak. The days were lengthening toward the summer solstice, and there was still peach-colored light along the western horizon, enough to illuminate the pathways through the gardens.

He watched for Meriel, but saw no pale fluttering silk to guide him. If she wasn't at the tree house, he'd never find her.

When he reached the clearing that held the oak, he paused to peruse the tree house. In the late twilight, the domed and minareted structure looked like a dream that had floated from an opium pipe and lodged in the solid branches of the ancient tree.

The ladder had been raised, so she was safely up in her castle. As he watched, he saw a glow of light suddenly illuminate one of the casement windows. There were matching windows on three sides of the tree house, and they were large enough to admit a man. It was time to see if he'd retained any of his boyhood climbing skill.

At the base of the oak, he peeled off his tightly fitted coat and tossed it aside to free up his arms. Then he studied the tree. The lowest branch was well above his head, but with a running start, he might be able to jump high enough to reach it.

He backed up, then sprinted forward and leaped upward. His fingers just missed the branch. Another try, and this time his clawing nails scrabbled across the bark.

Hurling himself into the air, he succeeded on his third try. The bark rough against his palms, he clambered onto the branch. From there, the climb to a branch level with the tree house was easy, though he was still ten feet or so away.

He looked into the open casement and saw Meriel pouring a grainy mixture into a small brass brazier. Her expression was cool and unyielding as marble, and he wondered briefly if it might be better to allow time for her temper to fade. No, he'd come this far, and he'd not retreat now. If he did, he might not be able to locate her again.

After a careful calculation of the distance, he launched himself at a high branch about halfway between his perch and the window. He caught it, then swung feet first through the open window. If Meriel liked grand entrances, this should appeal to her.

He landed hard and let himself drop into a crouch. She stopped dead, and her head snapped up as she stared at him.

As he straightened, he scanned his surroundings. The tree house was not a child's playhouse but a twelve-foot square Oriental palace with whitewashed walls and a floor layered with Persian carpets in jewel-rich colors. The wall next to the tree trunk was covered with book and storage shelves, while a padded bench ran the length of the wall opposite him. Embroidered pillows were mounded carelessly on the bench, spilling to the floor in luxuriant profusion.

His gaze returned to Meriel. With her flaxen hair and shimmering sari, she was as exotic as her setting. *Her hair was long, her foot was light, / And her eyes were wild.*

As calmly as if this were a normal occasion, he said, "You're furious at what my father said, and I don't blame you. Would you believe me if I told you that I'm really not a fortune hunter, intent only on plundering your inheritance?"

270

Ostentatiously ignoring him, she kindled the mixture in the brazier. A plume of musky, sweet-smelling smoke arose. Incense. He felt as if he had been transported to a land far, far from England. Or perhaps to a place of dreams.

Stepping to the bookcase, he chose a volume at random. It was a handwritten garden journal by one of Meriel's ancestors. "No wonder you keep this place private. Anyone visiting here would see how much more there is to you than what you allow the world to see."

She crossed to the window where he'd entered, and closed the casements. Then she pulled shut the heavy draperies that hung on each side. She did the same for the other windows, enclosing them in an intimate, private space.

Despite her air of nonchalance, he wasn't surprised when she suddenly dived across the room and snatched up a small rug. Underneath was the hatch, with the ladder coiled neatly between a pair of wooden railings that stretched from hatch to wall.

He caught her before she could unlatch the bolt that secured the hatch, his hand coming down over hers. Kneeling on the other side of the hatch, he said intensely, "You have nothing to fear from me, Meriel. Your uncle and my father have tried to arrange a marriage for you, but I will never do anything that is against your will."

Her gaze was enigmatic, not angry. Relieved, he said, "I hope that you know something of me by now. I am not my father. His opinions are not mine."

Her hand was warm beneath his, her face was only a hand span away. He could smell the heady fragrance of rose rising from her pearly skin.

As his pulse quickened, he wondered why the devil he had felt so compelled to pursue her when she fled the dinner table. It would be no bad thing if his father's crude remarks had persuaded her to reject marriage to Kyle. But he hated the thought that she might believe that *he* was interested only in her property.

Damnation, even he was having trouble separating himself from his brother. It would be fine if she thought ill of Kyle—but he wanted her to think well of Dominic the Deceitful. The time had come to explain who he was.

But it was hard to think when she was so near, her great eyes fixed on his face. His hand took on a life of its own, skimming up her bare arm to her shoulder. Under his palm, her skin was silken smooth, pulsing with life. He whispered, "Meriel."

Her lips parted, and she leaned forward until they met his. He pulled her into a drugging kiss, intoxicated by her nearness, her scent, the taste and welcome of her mouth. *This* was why he had come, because he hungered and thirsted for her.

Under the thin layers of silk, he felt curves unfettered by corset or whalebone. He slid one hand down her back, under the sari, feeling the lithe flex of her spine. She was like a steel butterfly, fragile and strong at the same time.

The increasing discomfort of an erection straining against tight trousers forcibly reminded him how wrong this was. He must be responsible not only for himself, but for her. Releasing Meriel, he sat back on his heels and said unsteadily, "This is not wise, Meriel. I cannot claim to care for you and then commit an act that will have consequences far beyond a night of pleasure."

Getting to his feet, he offered her a hand up. She rose lightly, making no attempt to mask her desire. The sensual tension that had been building since the beginning thrummed between them, taut and unmistakable. He felt as if he were splitting into pieces, his rational, responsible side saying this was madness while the rest of him—blood, heart, sinew—clamored that the love and tenderness he felt could not be wrong.

Scented smoke had filled the room, clouding his judgment. What the devil was in that incense? Realizing that he must leave before it was too late, he knelt by the hatch and slid open the bolt. Then he pulled on the inset handle. The hatch didn't move. He tugged again. Nothing.

Then he noticed the key lock and realized that it could be turned from either side. Meriel had used both key and bolt to preserve her privacy. Or had she guessed that he would come, and wanted to make it difficult for him to leave? His increasingly hazy mind could not decide.

He stood again with the vague idea of leaving the way he had come, even if it meant risking his neck, but Meriel stood between him and the window. No longer avoiding his eyes, she held his gaze as she unclasped the golden brooch that had secured her sari. After tossing it aside, she tugged at the free end of the silk that draped over her shoulder and down her back.

He stood paralyzed while she began unwinding the garment. The silence was absolute, except for the chime of her bangle bracelets and his rough breath.

As each layer of translucent silk fell away, her body became more visible. An ivory goddess, more perfect than mortal man dared imagine.

The last layer of silk slipped sensuously from her body and pooled around her feet, leaving her clad only in shining hair, golden jewelry, and provocative mehndi that cupped her small breasts and encircled her navel before arrowing toward her thighs with blatant provocation. Helplessly he realized that no man could resist such loveliness, not when it was coupled with the incendiary craving he saw in her eyes. He was certain now that she had expected him to come to her, and prepared accordingly.

Two steps brought her slim body against him. As he tried to force his muscles to retreat, she drew him into an ardent, open-mouthed kiss.

Resistance shattered. Feverishly he caressed her, blood hammering in his temples so fiercely that he was barely aware of her hands clawing at his clothing, of how together they stripped away his garments until bare flesh pressed against bare flesh.

As breath roughened and knees weakened, she tugged him down to the thickly carpeted floor, laughing with giddy triumph. "La Belle Dame Sans Merci," the beauty without mercy who could steal a man's soul, and make him grateful for the loss.

He came down full length beside her, his mouth devouring as it traveled from throat to softly curving breasts. As he stroked over the gentle arc of her belly, her lips separated and she began to croon a plaintive, emotion-saturated melody. At first her song was so soft it might have been imagined, but as he explored more boldly, the tone strengthened until her rib cage vibrated like a purring cat's.

The haunting sound penetrated his passion-hazed mind, reminding him of issues beyond the hot urgency of the moment. Raising his head, he said huskily, "Speak to me, Meriel. Tell me you truly understand the meaning of what we are doing."

Her darkened lashes lifted, revealing eyes of blind, unfocused green, but her breathy song did not shape into words. He slid one hand between her thighs. They separated with inviting ease. Gently he caressed the moist, sensitive folds of hidden flesh. She shivered, and her crooning ended as she gasped for breath.

Her uninhibited passion was irresistible, but

a stab of insight warned that if she could satisfy her needs without revealing herself, she might spend the rest of her life barricaded in her private world. Her desire was the most potent weapon he had for calling forth the whole of her complex, entrancing nature. "Please, say my name," he urged again. "Or even the single word 'yes'..."

She closed her eyes, rejecting his plea even as her nails curled into his back.

Damning himself for a fool, he said hoarsely, "I will not continue unless I hear you ask in your own voice. If you will not trust me, we should not be together."

Again, she offered no words, only restless, questing hands.

He broke from her embrace and pushed himself up with one arm. Then he gazed at her, aching. She was his heart's desire, as alluring and dangerous as Keats's fairy queen. "I'm sorry, my love," he whispered. "So sorry."

Then he started to rise, while he was still strong enough to do the right thing.

Chapter 25

Her eyes flew open in disbelief. No, he could not stop now, or she would burst into fatal flame.

The light around him flared crimson with desire, but his muscles flexed as he pushed himself upright. She realized with deep, twisting pain that he truly did mean to abandon her.

She could not bear for him to go, even if his price was the private world that had sheltered her so well.

She caught his wrist desperately. "No!" Though singing had kept her voice healthy, it was an effort to shape words after so many years of not speaking. Haltingly she said, "Please. Don't. Go."

His expression changed in an instant from haggard determination to a warmth that hurt to behold. "Oh, Meriel," he whispered. "My dearest one."

He enfolded her, warming her with kisses as he resumed the caresses that had driven her to the edge of madness. She sucked in her breath as jagged sensations ripped through her veins. Her hips moved with increasing frenzy until she could bear no more. She convulsed, her whole body shuddering out of control. He held her, keeping her safe even as she spun into a place she had never been before.

She was still quivering with aftershocks when he braced himself between her legs. She opened her eyes, drinking in the sight of him. Ah, but he was splendid, broad of shoulder, hard of muscle, her mehndi branding his skin. At long last, her mate.

The taut lines around his eyes showed how much it cost him to enter slowly instead of thrusting like a maddened stallion. She arched against him, realizing with dazed wonder that this was the difference between man and beast, this tenderness more devastating than passion.

He filled her, stretching her flesh in a startling but not unpleasant way. The searing intimacy was everything she had yearned for, the melding of two bodies into one—and the fervent need to give back what she had received. She rocked against him and was shocked to feel once more the rising tide of desire.

He gasped and began thrusting uncontrollably, the force of his movements driving them crazily across the carpet until they were against the divan. She clung to him, her limbs locking around his back and hips as he penetrated not only her body but her soul, filling her with radiance, driving out the shadows that had haunted her for a lifetime.

He cried out and went rigid, violent tremors racking him as he spilled his seed within her. Once more she spun into madness, and learned that fulfillment was even greater when they tumbled into the abyss in each other's arms.

As passion ebbed, he held her close. Blood and spirit and breath returned to normal. And with sanity came the bleak necessity of facing the new land into which she had been reborn.

Peace. Contentment. Love. He lay on his side, dreamily caressing her back as she hid her face in his shoulder, her shining hair spilling every which way. He felt a sense of wonder that she had finally dared to speak, dissolving the last barrier between them. Though he admitted wryly that words could not begin to describe such wonders as what had just passed between them.

Their sweat-slicked bodies were cooling in the evening air, so he pulled a folded blanket off the bench above and tucked it around them both. How long would they be able to savor this precious, simple closeness before they must deal with the fact that Pandora's box had been opened, and could never be closed again?

Not long, for as he settled down again he realized that she was quietly crying. Alarmed, he brushed the heavy hair from her face so that he could see her expression. "What's wrong, Meriel? Did I hurt you?"

She shook her head, and hid her face again.

"Then why are you crying as if your heart is breaking?" he murmured against her temple. She felt so fragile as he held her. His contentment vanished as he berated himself for allowing passion to overwhelm judgment. "Tell me what's wrong, sweeting. Now that you've proved you can talk, I want to hear everything you have to say."

Her voice a husky whisper, she said, "I had not known...how lonely I was."

Her words tore at his heart. He'd wanted her to become vulnerable to him, and now that she was, he could scarcely bear it. Tenderly, he brushed the tears from her cheeks. "You'll never have to be lonely again, not as long as I live."

She sighed a little, not convinced. Realizing uneasily that he had just made a sweeping promise that he might be unable to fulfill, he changed the subject. "You've never spoken to anyone else, not even Kamal?"

"No need." She rolled from his embrace onto her back, saying with tart humor, "Kamal does not plague me as you do."

He grinned. "I assume that even though people spoke in front of you as if you were a piece of furniture, you've always understood everything around you."

She shrugged. "When I listened."

He suspected that she had ignored the world more often than not. "When you paid attention, I imagine that you learned much more than anyone gave you credit for."

Her lips curved into a faint smile. "Perhaps."

He could see the effort it took for her to use language after so many years without speaking. If not for her wordless songs, her voice might have withered away altogether. "I can see that you intend to be a woman of few words."

She slanted a wicked glance. "You talk enough for two."

He laughed. "With you silent, I had to. Until now." He propped his head up on his hand, his gaze on her face. "Why have you deliberately cut yourself off from normal human interactions? You were very young when you made that decision."

"It was not like that," she said slowly. "The fire, the slaughter, the captivity, were more than I could bear." Her eyes closed for a moment as pain spasmed across her face. "In my mind I came back to Warfield, ignoring the zenana as much as possible. It was not until long after I returned home I started to turn outward again. By then, I had lost the habit of speech. And...I liked my life as it was. I had everything I wanted. Speaking—being considered normal—would have changed that."

"And you did not want change."

She did not bother to reply. He studied her delicate profile, seeing the sensitive child who had gone through hell and had only gradually begun to heal after returning to her beloved home. It was easy to understand why she hadn't wished to trade a comfortable life with great freedom for the dubious advantages of "normal" existence. His own sister had railed at the confines of ladylike restrictions more than once.

But Meriel's yearnings for passion and closeness were bringing change whether she wanted it or not. It was time to begin clearing the air. "Were you listening when Lord Maxwell first came to Warfield?"

"Kyle Renbourne. Viscount Maxwell." Her eyes glinted. "A major prize in the Marriage Mart."

One of the ladies must have used that term. He smiled, but only briefly, for the reminder of Kyle was sobering. He had been torn between loyalty to his brother and to Meriel. Now his reckless selfindulgence meant that he was irrevocably committed to her, and Kyle would never forgive him. Burying his pain at that thought for later, he said bluntly, "I'm not Lord Maxwell."

Her gaze sharpened. "Not Renbourne?"

"Yes, but Dominic Renbourne, not Kyle. I'm

Lord Maxwell's twin brother." He grimaced. "I'm not proud of this, Meriel. Since we look enough alike to fool people who don't know us well, Kyle asked me to take his place so he could be elsewhere. Though I didn't want to, he was...persuasive. I thought coming to Warfield would be a simple matter. I would say little, let you become accustomed to me— or rather, someone who looked like me. Then leave."

Catching her gaze, he said intensely, "I didn't expect to fall in love with you, but I have. That changes everything."

To his relief, she didn't recoil in horror, but neither did she declare love for him as he had secretly hoped. Instead, she regarded him with coolly assessing eyes. "So. No wonder you seemed different. More dangerous."

"Me, dangerous?" he said, genuinely startled. "Kyle can be an awkward devil, but I've always had an easy disposition."

Ignoring that, she said, "Kyle is a hard name, all edges. I like Dominic better."

"Good. I hope you like Dominic well enough to marry me, since I have well and truly compromised you." He took her hand. "Though I'm not the prize in the Marriage Mart my brother is, I do love you. I hope that's good enough."

She drew away and sat up. One end of the sari lay within reach, so she pulled the fabric loosely around her, though the sheer silk emphasized rather than concealed her nakedness. "Such a passion you have for marriage. I do not share it."

A chill went through him. He should have known that speech would not instantly resolve all differences. "Only wedded couples are supposed to behave as we have."

Her brows arched with disbelief. "You have never mated before?"

"I have known other women, but none like you."

Her eyes narrowed. "None so rich?"

His jaw tightened. She had picked up a great deal of cynicism in her overheard conversations. "None has been so rich," he agreed, "but it is not your wealth that draws me, Meriel. I would gladly marry you even if you were penniless."

She cocked her head to one side, the golden earrings swinging with a faint, teasing *tching*. "You have a fortune?"

"No," he said steadily. "A small independent income, but not a fortune."

"So your brother, who is rich, wishes to marry me for my money, while you, who are poor, do not." She injected an unnerving amount of disbelief into her voice.

He sighed. "This is a question that must be answered by faith, not proof, sprite. You either believe me or you don't."

Her mouth twisted. "And what do I know of men? How can I judge?"

"You can listen to your heart," he said quietly.

"My heart says that change is coming too

quickly." Her cynicism vanished, leaving stark discomfort. "For a woman, marriage means trusting her body and property wholly to the ownership of a man. When I was drawing mehndi on Jena Ames, she told me what had happened to her. Why should I risk that when I don't have to?"

Why indeed, if she didn't love or trust him. Fighting down his resentment at how easily she dismissed his declaration, he got to his feet and pulled on his trousers and shirt. The brazier had burned out, but heavily scented smoke still clouded the room, so he drew the draperies back from a window and opened the casements. Then he leaned out and filled his lungs with clean, damp air.

He thought back on the affairs he'd had. Though he'd never been a womanizer, he'd experienced his share of the delights of the flesh. He'd lain with randy widows, lusty maids, and sometimes bored wives. But he'd never been involved in a relationship where either party thought their liaison was anything more than a passing pleasure.

Until Meriel, where "till death do us part" seemed like the only possible outcome for the intimacies they had shared. Most gently bred young ladies would agree wholeheartedly, but she was not like anyone else. Not that he wanted her to become conventional at the price of her magical uniqueness—but marriage was one convention he dearly wished she would embrace.

The increasing clarity of his thoughts

reminded him of an earlier question. He turned, folding his arms over his chest. "What did you burn in the brazier?"

"Mostly frankincense." She began to braid her hair. "A little opium."

"My God, opium?" He stared at her. So that was why his thoughts had been scrambled, and his sorely tried willpower had finally snapped. "How could you?"

She shrugged. "You were so stubborn. Strong measures were required."

Her casualness was a forceful reminder of how *different* she was. She truly did not see the outrageousness of her behavior. Wanting to make her understand, he asked dryly, "What would you think of a man who used strong drink to seduce a lady?"

Her eyes narrowed. "Despicable."

So she had learned at least some morality from her guardians. "Is it any more right that you used a drug to persuade me to do something against my will?"

She froze, her braiding hands still. "You seemed willing to me."

"My body certainly was," he said sharply. "But my conscience forbade sexual intimacy because it would be *wrong*. Though it wasn't easy, I had managed to behave honorably—until you saw fit to drug me."

Her face tightened. "Why do you think our mating was wrong?"

"Because you are betrothed to my brother, not me." He frowned, seeking the right words. "And even more because no man of honor

285

should take advantage of a young woman whose judgment is impaired. Such behavior is beneath contempt."

Her eyes narrowed to feline slits. "You think me mad?"

"Not mad. But your upbringing has been so unusual that you cannot fully understand society's dictates, and why they should be obeyed."

She resumed her braiding. "Your honor is safe, Renbourne. I was the evil seducer, not you."

He made an impatient gesture with his hand. "What matters is not blame, but consequences." He hesitated, realizing he must ask an awkward question, not only to satisfy his own curiosity, but because the answer could make a difference in their situation. "Have you ever...lain with another man?"

She sighed, her anger draining away. "No, though I was not virgin. In the zenana, there was talk of giving me to a neighboring rajah as a concubine. My hair made me a great novelty, and it is not unknown for small girls to become brides in India. Concerned because I was so little, one of the older women, Asma, used a stone lingam to remove my maidenhead."

He would not have understood if he hadn't seen a lingam during his school days. The son of an Indian army officer had produced one to impress his classmates, and the boys had passed around the crudely carved male organ with fascination and nervous laughter. He was appalled to think of a delicate child being subjected to such a barbaric ritual. "How horrible for you."

"It was kindly meant, to spare me undue suffering." She crossed her arms on her drawn-up knees and rested her head on them, hiding her face. "Asma was whipped for tampering with me, and it was decided that I should be given back to the English. Perhaps Asma foresaw that might happen."

He could only dimly grasp how alien her experiences had been. No wonder she was frank about subjects that would make a more sheltered girl swoon, or that she had returned to her own people permanently altered. Trying to be as matter-of-fact as she, he said, "Despite the lingam, you were a virgin, which means that marriage is the proper course. Would that be so bad? I had thought you cared for me."

Her eyes softened, for he hadn't quite managed to keep emotion from his voice. "You know I do, but that doesn't mean I want marriage." She gazed at him pleadingly. "Can't we stay as we are? These last weeks have been so happy."

He sighed. "That's not possible, sprite. This visit is courtship intended to lead to marriage. The world would be horrified if we chose to live together unwed. Your guardians would never permit it, even if I'm willing to be seen as a seducer of innocence, which I am not. If we don't marry, I must leave."

Her jaw set stubbornly. "I am Lady of Warfield. How dare anyone censure me!"

Shades of her medieval ancestors. History

books and ancient journals lined her book-shelves, and had obviously affected her thinking. "This is the world we must live in, Meriel. If you were a widow of mature years, you could offer me some post such as business manager and we could be together if we were discreet about it. But you are young and beautiful and thought to be disordered in your wits, which is very different."

She scowled. "That is not just."

"Perhaps not, but the time has come to pay the price for your years of doing exactly what you wanted and letting the world think you mad," he said bluntly. "Even though you are now speaking, it will take time for your family to accept you as a sane, intelligent woman capable of making her own decisions."

She drew her sari more closely, like a shawl. "I will talk only to you."

He almost groaned with exasperation. How could she be so intelligent and so blind at the same time? "You can't just pretend nothing has happened. If necessary, I'll tell the ladies that you can speak as well as they do."

"They won't believe that unless they hear me with their own ears."

He bit off an oath, knowing she was right. If he claimed that she talked to him without offering proof, the ladies would think *his* wits were disordered.

"You may want to deny change, but what if you are with child? It's possible, and pregnancy is not something that can be ignored. If you bear a baby outside of marriage, it would be a social outcast because of our immoral behavior. Would you want that?"

She gasped and laid a hand on her belly, as if she had not considered the possibility. He had a brief, crazed vision of her choosing to marry Kyle, then bearing Dominic's son as heir to Wrexham. That would certainly be a younger son's vengeance for the injustice of fate.

Wrapping her arms around her knees again, she began to rock like a distraught child. He swore at himself for upsetting her. Even more, for letting this situation develop. The opium couldn't have affected him if he'd had the sense to stay away from her.

He left the window and knelt beside her, petting her bare arm comfortingly. "I'm sorry for alarming you, sprite. If you aren't with child—and probably you're not—your life can stay just as it is now. I will leave, and you'll forget me soon." Though he was painfully aware that he would not forget her.

"No!" Her head whipped up, and she stared at him. "Can't you be my business manager? I can be as discreet as any old widow."

The idea was dangerously tempting. To be with Meriel without incurring the wrath of his family, or the rest of the world...but it wasn't possible. "That's not good enough, Meriel. I want us to hold our heads up before God and country, not hide in the shadows like adulterers."

"It shouldn't matter what others think!" she said passionately.

She had the soul of an aristocrat, or a democrat, he wasn't sure which. "Unless you live alone in a cave, other people's opinions matter." He caught her gaze, wanting to impress her with his words. "The choice is yours, Meriel. You can refuse to marry anyone, and have your life of freedom. Or you can marry me." He swallowed hard. "Or Kyle, or some other man. But I will not be your illicit lover."

She closed her eyes, as if she could block out his words. With her hair pulled back and the skin taut over her cheekbones, she no longer looked like a child. She was a woman, and tired. "I don't want you to go," she whispered. "But I...I need time to accept so many changes. Will you not grant me that?"

"We have a little time, until my brother returns from his journey." He opened his arms, and she leaned into his embrace. "Perhaps another fortnight. By then you might know whether or not you are with child."

Meriel sighed and rested her head against him. Overwhelmed with tenderness, he brushed a silken tendril of hair back from her temple. She was like a butterfly emerging from a chrysalis, horrendously vulnerable but determined to survive in a strange new world. He could only imagine how much courage that took.

He bent and gave her what was intended to be a comforting kiss. Her head tilted back and her lips molded to his. As he felt the first stirrings of arousal, he had a brief, fierce battle with his conscience. What was wrong earlier was wrong still, and this time he didn't have the excuse of opium to haze his judgment.

She slid one hand under his loose shirt. "At dinner, I liked knowing that beneath your gentleman's garb, you wear my mehndi on your skin."

As her fingers fluttered teasingly across his chest, his resolve wavered. Their situation could hardly be worsened from what it was now. And gods above, he wanted so much to make love to her, body and soul, to show her the depth of his caring.

He pulled the sari from her shoulder and kissed the graceful henna lines that curved around her breasts. The designs were so primitive, so un-English. They made it easier to forget the world of rules and strictures that lay outside their sanctuary.

With his tongue, he began to trace the mehndi down her body, tasting the faint salt of her skin as he inhaled the intoxicating fragrance of rose perfume. Her choked gasps were the richest of aphrodisiacs.

This time when they came together, both were fully aware of what they did.

Meriel had decided to sleep in the tree house, to avoid the leave-taking of Wrexham and Lucia in the morning. Dominic would have liked to stay with her, but better not to draw attention to his whereabouts during the night. He drew her into one last kiss before descending the ladder, murmuring, "Sleep well, sprite."

291

"I'll dream of you," she said with a soft laugh. "Dominic."

It was the first time she had called him by his given name. Hearing the word on her lips made departure feel as if he were chopping off a vital part of himself.

Even worse was walking alone through the night, haunted by a terrible fear that never again would they be so close.

Chapter 26

As Lucia hugged Dominic, she said under her breath, "Well done, Dom. You look so stern this morning, I almost thought you really were Kyle."

He grinned as he released her. "Try to behave yourself, little sister."

She widened her eyes with mock innocence, then turned to offer effusive farewells to her hostesses. Guests and ladies were gathered beside the Wrexham coach, with the Warfield residents uniformly eager to see the earl go. As the departure rituals were observed, Dominic gave silent thanks that no one had mentioned the awkwardness of the previous evening's dinner.

His gratitude was premature. After formally thanking the ladies for their hospitality, his father turned to him. Keeping his voice down, he asked, "Did you catch that little minx and give her a lesson in courtesy last night?"

For a paralyzed moment, Dominic's mind played pictures of the lessons actually learned. Collecting himself, he answered, "I explained the need to conform to society's expectations. I believe my words may have had some effect."

"I hope so." The earl shook his head, his expression troubled. "I don't hesitate to say that I am having grave doubts about this marriage. I know Amworth said the girl was normal once, but she certainly isn't now. I can't see her as the Countess of Wrexham, nor the mother of a future earl. Perhaps the betrothal should be ended."

Dominic felt a surge of pure fury. How *dare* his father treat Meriel first as a rich orphan to be exploited, then as a madwoman with no value or feelings? Barely in time, he reined in his anger and said in his flattest voice, "For me to withdraw from the betrothal would be a grave breach of honor."

"Yes, but all along the understanding has been that the girl must be willing. Surely you can persuade her to change her mind." The earl gave a raucous laugh. "See that a handsome stableboy is hired. One lusty enough to hold her attention so you can bow out gracefully."

"You appall me, sir," Dominic said icily.

The earl squinted at him nearsightedly. "Where is your humor, boy? You can't think I was serious. She may be mad, but she's a lady still. Deserves better than a stableboy, even if she isn't fit to be a countess."

Dominic swallowed, sensing that he was very close to giving himself away. "My apologies, sir. Lady Meriel inspires...protectiveness."

"Obviously," the earl grunted. "Do your best, Maxwell. I want no scandals, but I shan't weep if the girl decides against marriage."

Ironically, on this issue Wrexham and Meriel were in accord. "I have no more wish for scandal than you, sir," Dominic said woodenly. "Have a safe journey."

As he watched his father turn to the coach, Dominic felt a sudden, overwhelming urge to ask the question that had gnawed at him for half a lifetime. When he was younger, he hadn't dared ask, and in more recent years he hadn't had the opportunity. Using Kyle's inflections with extra care, he asked, "Why did you send my brother and me to different schools?"

Wrexham halted, frowning. "Why the devil do you ask that now?"

"I've always wondered." Which was true, even if little else Dominic had said today was the truth.

"You were too close to each other. If you'd gone to Eton together, you'd have ended up with only one life between you," the earl said gruffly. "That would have been bad for you, and worse for your brother. You needed to be separated while you were still young enough to make other friends."

Dominic's lips thinned as he thought of the misery he'd endured the first terms at his school. "Did it ever occur to you how painful that would be?"

Weary regret showed in his father's cataract-hazed eyes. "How could I not know, the way the two of you carried on? Your brother never forgave me, and I've often suspected that you haven't, either. But I was right to do it. Even your mother agreed." With a curt nod, he climbed inside the coach and settled onto the velvet-covered seat.

Lucia bounced in after him in a flurry of laughter and billowing skirts. The earl's face relaxed into the smile that he reserved for her alone. His daughter had never given him the trouble his sons had.

A footman closed the door, cutting off Dominic's sight of his family, and the coach started down the long driveway. He stood beside the ladies, mechanically waving good-bye as his thoughts churned.

His mother had agreed to the separation? That was news; he'd assumed that it was done over her objections because she had wept for her sons' parting. But she was a warmhearted woman, and could have wept for their misery while agreeing that separation was for the best. She'd died not long after his departure.

To his shock, he realized that he had to concede that his father had been right to separate them. When it happened he'd felt only the pain, but by the time he entered the army, he'd reached the same conclusion as Wrexham: that he must build an independent life, out of his brother's shadow.

It was hard to admit that the earl was right. Even harder was accepting that his harsh, domineering father had acted from genuine concern rather than casual cruelty.

How could things be so much the same, yet utterly changed? For three days, Meriel and Renbourne had gone on morning rides and worked in the gardens together, usually under the amiable eye of Kamal. Yet everything was...different. Meriel no longer burned with vague, unfocused lust; now that she knew what it was like to join her body with his, passion was deeper and far more compelling.

They were pruning the topiary again; it was a job that never ended. She knelt beside one of the hounds so that she could shape the outstretched paws. Feeling Renbourne's gaze, she glanced up and saw that he was watching her, his eyes grave.

Softly, so that Kamal wouldn't hear, she whispered, "Dominic."

His face lit up with a smile of dazzling intimacy. She caught her breath, wanting to pull him down to the fragrant turf and swarm all over him, biting and rolling and kissing until they were covered in grass stains and he was thrusting into her, his eyes blind with need and his heart hammering against hers.

Instead, pulse pounding, she lowered her gaze and chopped off an unruly sprig of yew. For three days she'd thought of him constantly, battling the temptation to seduce him out of his good intentions. She doubted that he would reject her if she slipped into his bed at night.

But she had controlled her impulses, rather to her surprise. Though she did not agree with his position, it would be very bad to tempt him to betray his notions of honor. Wryly she recognized a significant change—she was behaving with maturity. Being an irresponsible madwoman was simpler, and much more amusing.

Luckily she had soon learned that she was not with child. She knew little of babies, and was certainly not ready to face the complications pregnancy would bring.

She sighed. For years she'd been quite content with her life, reveling in armloads of blossoms, and fertile soil between her toes, and nature's glorious, ever-changing panorama. Now contentment had been supplanted by a hunger for a man in her bed.

But the man wished to wed, and gratifying her desires would come only at a terrifyingly high price. She'd had nightmares every night since their tryst, waking with pounding heart and fragmentary memories of fire and screams and pain. There was no mystery about the dreams; they represented her terror of the outside world she had fled.

Would it be possible to marry and still stay safe at Warfield? Or would there be ever-increasing pressures to "take her place in the world"? To be Lady Meriel, heiress of Warfield, with a London town house and a presentation at court? Ever since arriving, Renbourne had been hell-bent on persuading her to try new ventures. She hadn't minded in the case of riding, but leaving Warfield was quite a different matter.

She slanted a glance at Renbourne, who was stretching up to prune the head of a leaping topiary horse. Such lovely long, taut muscles. He gave her joy unlike any she had ever known. She even trusted him—to a point.

But the nightmares had come with flames and dark, unintelligible messages of betrayal. Why, she didn't understand, but over the years wariness had become part of her. Though she trusted Renbourne as a lover, even her lust-addled heart could not quite make the leap to trusting her life and Warfield to his hands.

And without that trust, there could be no marriage.

Dominic accepted a sherry from Mrs. Marks with a quip, then glanced at the doorway to see if Meriel had arrived for dinner. Four days had passed since they'd made love, and the time had dragged like four years. The night before, he'd woken sweating from a fevered dream of intimately twined bodies, and barely restrained himself from going through the moonlit corridor to her room.

As promised, Meriel had continued silent, except for an occasional flick of words meant for his ears alone. He wondered if she recognized that each time she did that, he was stricken with paralyzing lust that faded with excruciating slowness.

Yet tormenting though it was to be near her all day without touching, it was better than not seeing her at all. Uneasily he was aware that time was running out. He would wait two or three days more before asking Meriel if she was coming to terms with the idea of marriage. Several times he'd caught her regarding him wistfully, as if he were only a memory. That didn't bode well, for he would have to leave if she still refused to marry him.

He heard a sound outside the salon, not Meriel's light footsteps but the heavy strides of a grown man. The butler? No, too solid and arrogant. Probably a visitor; he'd never seen such a house for people arriving unannounced. Still, he'd survived Amworth and Wrexham, so he should be all right.

A travel-stained man of middle years swept into the room, shadowed by two equally travel-stained footmen, who silently took position against the wall. Tall and powerfully built, the newcomer carried himself like a soldier. His furious gaze raked over the three people in the salon. "What is the meaning of this?"

"We are gathering for dinner, Lord Grahame," Mrs. Marks said mildly. "How nice that you are in time to join us."

Dominic froze. Gods above, it only needed this! But what the devil was Grahame doing in England? He wasn't due back from the Continent for weeks.

Echoing his thoughts, Mrs. Rector chimed in, "Such an unexpected pleasure. We thought you were still in France."

"Don't insult me with pleasantries. I am gravely disappointed in you both." Grahame glowered at the women. "I decided to return home early when I received news of Amworth's illness. Imagine my shock when I visited the Warfield solicitor in London to learn Amworth's condition, and discovered what has been going on behind my back. The solicitor has been disquieted by this...this marriage plot, and was grateful for the chance to tell me all about it."

He turned his scowl on Dominic. "I presume that you are Viscount Maxwell. Is your reputation so vile that no normal heiress will have you?"

Meriel appeared in the doorway behind Grahame. Her eyes widened as she took in the scene at a glance. Then she vanished in a swirl of blue skirts. He was grateful for that, because the confrontation unfolding was going to be very, very ugly.

Hoping calm might defuse some of the tension, he said, "Lord Amworth explained to me how you and he both wish only the best for your niece, but disagree about how to achieve that. Having become well acquainted with Lady Meriel, I agree entirely with Lord Amworth: she is well suited to marriage. I'm grateful that Amworth chose to honor a long-standing plan to unite our families."

"Very prettily said," Grahame growled. "But pretty words won't disguise the fact that taking advantage of a mentally deficient girl is the action of a scoundrel."

"You underestimate your niece's abilities," Dominic said, still calm. "She is not in the common way, but there is nothing wrong with her wits or her judgment. And ultimately, the decision to marry is hers."

Grahame's fists clenched furiously. "Nonsense! As one of her guardians, I have the obligation and authority to prevent any ill-advised liaison. That is why Amworth tried to hustle my niece into marriage while I was away."

"*Do* you have the authority?" Dominic retorted. "Meriel is of age, and I believe that no court has ever declared her unfit."

"That can be arranged!" Grahame's eyes narrowed. "I'll grant that Amworth meant well, but if I take this matter to court, any judge would agree that the girl needs protection, not to be handed over to a fortune hunter."

"One really can't call Maxwell a fortune hunter, Lord Grahame," Mrs. Rector said unexpectedly. "His breeding and station are equal to Meriel's, and his kindness and perception make him an ideal husband for a young woman of her...delicate nature. Lord Amworth chose well."

Grahame stared at Mrs. Rector, who accepted his hard gaze with her usual placidity. What a splendid old girl she was, Dominic thought fondly. She looked soft and sweet as marzipan, but she had the courage to stand up to a raging earl.

Suppressing a guilty pang that he was not the desirable heir to Wrexham but the much less desirable younger son, he said, "I respect your care for Lady Meriel, sir, but I believe you know her less well than you think."

Grahame gave him a look of utter contempt. "In a matter of days, you've become an expert on the girl, while I, who have cared for her since she was a child, know nothing? Such arrogance!"

"She has grown and changed even in the short time I have known her." Dominic made a swift decision. "So much so that she has begun to talk."

Grahame's jaw dropped, and both of the ladies inhaled in shock. Grahame rallied first. "Is this true, Mrs. Marks?"

"It's the first I've heard of it," she replied, wide-eyed. "Meriel has really spoken, Lord Maxwell?"

"Yes, and very intelligently, too. So far, she has been too shy"—it was as good an explanation as any—"to talk to anyone but me, but I believe that in time she will converse as freely as you or I."

The older man snorted. "I will believe that when I hear her with my own ears."

Doubting that Meriel would talk to this group even to save him from looking like a liar, Dominic replied, "As I said, she is shy. It isn't easy for her to change her relationship to the world. She must be allowed to progress at her own speed."

"It sounds to me as if you've invented a parcel of lies to cover up your shameless greed." Grahame's mouth twisted. "I wish to God

that Meriel *could* speak. I would give anything to hear her call me 'Uncle' again, but
she never will. She is incapable of understanding even the simplest of comments or
requests."

Dominic felt a flash of irritation at the
older man's obduracy, but as he knew from
personal experience, Meriel's fragile beauty
inspired protectiveness. Her uncle was showing
perfectly reasonable concern. His tone conciliatory, he pointed out, "She doesn't always
pay attention to what people say, but she has
a masterful knowledge of gardening. The
mehndi she paints require intelligence, skill,
and talent. Every hour I have spent in her company has given more proof of a fine, unconventional mind."

"I've often thought she understands more
than we realize," Mrs. Marks agreed.

"You believe that because you wish to
believe it. Just as you think well of Maxwell
because he's a personable young man, and you
want to think well of him." Grahame frowned
at Dominic. "But how can you bear the
thought of an innocent child being given to a
man of the world who will despoil and abandon
her?"

"Meriel is *not* a child!" Dominic said vehe-
mently. "She's a woman—and she deserves to
be treated like one."

Grahame froze when he heard the passion
in Dominic's voice. "My God, you've bedded
her, haven't you?" the older man gasped.
"You...you disgusting libertine!"

A moment too slowly, Dominic protested, "I swear that I have not seduced Lady Meriel." But she had seduced him, and his guilt at allowing that made his denial sound feeble and unconvincing. Even his advocate, Mrs. Rector, looked upset.

Exploding across the room, Grahame snarled, "I should demand satisfaction, but a duel would tarnish Meriel's reputation. You have half an hour to leave Warfield." His jaw worked, a muscle jumping under the skin. "And if you ever set foot here again, I swear before God I will kill you without the formality of a duel."

To his footmen, he ordered, "Accompany this swine to his room while he collects his things, then escort him and his servants from the estate. If he attempts to elude you, or to seek out Lady Meriel, stop him by any means necessary."

Grahame had come with the intention of throwing the interloper out, Dominic realized. That was why he'd brought two burly footmen. No wonder he hadn't listened to reason—his mind was already made up.

Dominic's frayed temper nearly snapped. Meriel was a woman grown, not a helpless doll without a mind or will of her own. This was her house, and he was quite sure that she wanted him to stay. Her uncle had no right to evict him.

And yet—by the standards of normal society, Grahame's edict was justified. His co-guardian had gone behind his back to do something Grahame violently disagreed with, and now the man had arrived at Warfield to find that his niece's chaperons had failed miserably at their job. In Grahame's place, Dominic would be equally enraged.

He glanced at the ladies, but there was no aid there. Mrs. Rector was regarding him with large, sorrowful blue eyes, while Mrs. Marks tugged at the bell rope, summoning Morrison down in the servants' hall.

With as much dignity as he could manage, Dominic said, "I love Meriel, and I believe that she loves me. I hope that when tempers have cooled, we can discuss this matter reasonably."

Grahame gave a bark of bitter laughter. "There is nothing reasonable about my niece. You fool, sending you away is as much for your good as well as hers! She has twice attacked me with a knife, and I know that she has assaulted others as well. Be grateful that when you sleep at night, you won't have to worry about her sliding a blade between your ribs."

Uneasily Dominic remembered how Meriel had gone after the poacher. If she'd had a knife, she could have caused a serious injury. Yet that was not madness, but understandable rage. She was *not* mad!

Grahame gestured for his footmen to come forward. They were matched in height and strength, and must cost Grahame a pretty penny in wages. Dominic couldn't fight them both even if he wanted to.

Expression rigid, he set his long-forgotten sherry glass down and stalked to the door. But before leaving, he paused to say, "Remember, the ultimate decision about marriage belongs to Meriel, and no one else."

Grahame shook his head with disgust. "Your wits are as lacking as hers."

Dominic marched up the stairs to his room, his mind churning. Though Grahame didn't really have the legal authority to forbid Dominic's presence at Warfield, practically speaking, Dominic had no choice but to leave. Even if he could evade the footmen and find Meriel, he could never ask her to elope. Warfield was her home, and her roots ran as deep as those of the ancient oak that sheltered the tree house.

His only hope was to go to Lord Amworth, whose authority was equal to Grahame's. With Amworth's backing, he would be able to return—*if* Amworth was still among the living, and strong enough to fight Grahame for Meriel's future.

She did not even have a chance to say good-bye.

Meriel had retreated to her room to escape the unpleasantness in the salon. She always avoided her uncle Grahame. Though his military days were long gone, he still tended to bark at everyone as if they were troops under his command.

Then she heard jangling harness. Idly she glanced out, thinking to see Grahame's carriage being taken around the house. Instead, a grim-faced Renbourne was driving his curricle away from the stables, valet by his side and his horse tethered behind.

Her heart seemed to freeze. He was leaving, and not voluntarily, or two large, stolid men in her uncle's livery would not be flanking the vehicle.

At the head of the driveway Renbourne reined in his horses and gazed up at the house, his expression taut. She waved frantically, but the long rays of the setting sun were reflecting from the windows and he couldn't see her.

Shaking, she watched him start the horses down the drive. Though he had warned that the world would not accept an irregular union between them, she had not believed how swift and merciless disapproval could be.

Dizzily she realized that she might never see him again. She had refused his offer of marriage, and now her uncle had driven him from Warfield. Would he ever return after that double rejection?

Her shock was driven out by fury. How *dare* her uncle send away her lover! She was mistress of Warfield, and he had no right to treat her like a child. Whirling, she left her room and raced down the stairs. She *had* been a child to run away rather than enter the salon. If she had been by Renbourne's side, they could not have made him leave.

She must go after him. Moonbeam? No, going to the stables for the mare would take too long. Better to go by foot. The driveway curved widely. If she ran straight to the gate, she should arrive there just before the curricle. Then she would bring Renbourne back and he could order her servants to send her uncle and his men away.

She was heading for the front door when her uncle emerged from the salon in front of her. The light around him was steely gray.

"How convenient," he said in a voice of unnatural gentleness. "I was just coming to look for you. Don't worry, Meriel, I will take care of you. Finally you can receive treatment that might help your madness. Even if that can't be cured, at least I can put a stop to your wanton behavior."

She stopped in her tracks, anger turning to fear as she saw the expression in his eyes. He looked...implacable.

As he advanced on her, she slowly began to back away, pulse pounding.

"Don't run, my dear, I won't hurt you." His voice rose on the last words as he made a sudden leap toward her. "Get her!"

She spun about. While her uncle held her attention, one of his men had crept up behind her, an open blanket in his hands. Panic swept through her. Frantically she swerved, barely escaping the servant's grab.

"Don't let the little hellcat escape! We'll never find her if she gets out of the house," her uncle snapped. "But don't injure her."

Unable to get past the servant, she changed direction again. But she was boxed in, her uncle on one side, the servant on the other, the wall behind. Beyond Grahame, she saw the horror-struck faces of the ladies as they watched from the doorway of the salon.

Desperately she bolted toward the salon, praying that the women would help her, but she could not escape her uncle's lunge. Catching her with huge, hard hands, he swung her around to face him. Near hysteria, she kicked and clawed at his eyes.

"Damnation!" he swore as he struggled to secure her wrists. "If your lover could see you now, he'd stop claiming you're sane!"

The servant swooped in and enveloped her in scratchy folds of blanket. Then he threw her to the marble floor, knocking her breathless.

"Don't hurt her!" Mrs. Rector called out anxiously.

"We won't." Grahame dropped to his knees and began to roll her in the blanket. Gasping for air, she made frenzied attempts to escape, but he was too large, too strong. He overpowered her, trapping her arms and legs so tightly that she couldn't move.

When he was done, he lifted her cocooned body in his arms, panting, "You're safe now, Meriel. I'm here to take care of you."

She began to scream.

Chapter 27

The air vibrated with the sound of church bells striking the noon hour. Great slow basses, swift small trebles, melodious middle ringers. In the darkened room, Kyle held Constancia's hand and wondered if Catholic cities had more bells, or did he just notice them more here because he spent so much time waiting, and listening?

It was easier to think of bells than of the end that was approaching too swiftly. The day before he'd visited the nearest church, wanting to make sure the priest was suitable and would come quickly when summoned. The men had conversed in French, the only language they had in common, and Kyle had been impressed by Father Joaquín's gentle spirituality. He'd hoped not to see the priest again so soon, but half an hour earlier a servant had gone to the church at Constancia's request.

She dozed now, her gaunt face serene. She was thin to the point of transparency, but still possessed a terrible, poignant beauty.

It would have been so much easier to hire nurses and leave Constancia to her fate, but that would be such an act of cowardice that Kyle could never have forgiven himself. He'd had to bring her to Spain and stay until the end, no matter how difficult it was for him. Perhaps enduring pain was what it meant to be a man. Dominic had endured soul-deep pain in the army, and it had given him a core of toughness that Kyle envied.

Even hundreds of miles away at Dornleigh when Waterloo was fought, Kyle had felt the shadows of his brother's anguish, and a crushing weight that existed only in his mind. He'd been sure Dominic was dead or mortally wounded because of the terrible premonition he'd experienced when Dominic chose to enter the army. He'd tried to change his brother's mind, and succeeded only in creating a blazing row. When Dominic left to join his regiment, Kyle had been half convinced they'd never see each other again.

After the battle, he'd traveled to London at top speed with the idea of continuing on to Belgium. But by the time he reached the capital, casualty lists were being posted, and he learned that Dominic was alive, and only slightly wounded.

Ashamed of the way he'd panicked, he decided not to go to Brussels, fearing that his brother might laugh at the unnecessary concern. Later he regretted the decision, because Waterloo had crystallized their estrangement. Though Dominic's body hadn't been broken beyond repair, his spirit had been profoundly affected. Kyle often wondered what had aged his brother from boy to man so quickly, but Dominic never told him.

Would it have made a difference if Kyle had gone to Belgium right after the battle? Maybe he and his brother might have become friends again instead of drifting so far apart that they could barely speak civilly. Perhaps his premonition had meant alienation rather than physical death. If so, it had come true.

Luckily, not long after that he'd met Constancia. At first she had been an excitement and a pleasure. Later, she became a necessity.

Now, he was losing her.

"Querido." Her lashes swept up, revealing dark eyes that seemed to see beyond the mortal world.

"The priest will be here soon," he said soothingly.

She fluttered her fingers in a feeble gesture of impatience. "It is you who concern me, not him. I worry about you, mi corazón."

His brows arched with surprise. "Why? I'm fine."

"Nonetheless, I worry." She gave him a ghost of a smile. "Will you be happy? Will you be wise? Will you become friends with your brother again?"

"Odd. I was just thinking of Dominic." He smiled wryly. "I can't vouch for happiness or wisdom, but I promise to try to mend my relationship with my brother."

"One can ask no more than to try." She closed her eyes, collecting her strength. "And what of this English girl of scattered wits? Are you content to marry her?"

He hadn't thought of Lady Meriel for days, so he dutifully called her to mind. He could scarcely remember her face. Fragile and fawn-like, her pale coloring was bland next to the dark beauty he loved in Constancia. Still, she was not unattractive, and there was something very vulnerable about her. The knowledge was curiously appealing.

"The marriage will suit me well, I believe," he said slowly. "The girl needs someone to look out for her."

Constancia sighed. "That is why I worry. There is more to marriage than being needed, querido. You are too young to settle for so little."

Stung, he said, "I have not been man enough for you?"

Her thin fingers tightened around his. "You know that is not what I meant. I simply want you to have the best in your future—a young girl of wisdom and kindness who will adore you, and make your heart sing."

He bent and kissed her forehead. "I have had the best, Constancia. I cannot expect that to happen again."

"*Diablo!*" she muttered, tears glinting in her eyes. "This is the end of my life, querido, not of yours. Promise me that after I am gone, you will live life to the fullest. You deserve nothing less."

Before he could reply, Teresa opened the door and the white-robed priest entered. He nodded to Kyle, but it was Constancia he addressed, speaking in swift Spanish.

Kyle silently withdrew to the corner of the room and watched the alien rituals. A confession, not that Constancia had sins on her soul, for she was the best woman he had ever known. Then the last rites, performed with oil and grave, melodious phrases.

He felt a curious detachment. Above Constancia's bed hung a grim crucifix, lovingly painted to display maximum blood and suffering. The complete un-Englishness of the scene both intrigued and repelled him. But to

Constancia, this villa echoed her childhood home, and gave her comfort. That was worth the long, expensive journey.

As the solemn priest finished the last rites, a stunning idea struck Kyle. How could he not have thought of this before? Stepping forward, he said in French, "Father Joaquín, can you marry Señorita de las Torres and me right now?"

Constancia gasped, "Kyle!"

The priest blinked behind his silver-rimmed spectacles. "That isn't necessary. Having received extreme unction, she is in a state of grace, no longer a sinner."

"She was never a sinner," Kyle said sharply. "And I wish to marry her not for God, but for her, and for me." His voice gentled as he asked in English, "Will you have me for a husband, my dearest Constancia?"

She looked at him helplessly. "It is not right for you to go to your young bride as a newly widowed man, mi corazón."

He crossed to the bed and took her hand. "What is between us has nothing to do with her, Constancia." He hesitated, surprised at how intensely he wanted this marriage. "I do not wish to force you, but I would be very pleased, and honored, if you would consent to be my wife."

For a dozen heartbeats, she was silent. Then her lips curved into a slow, luminescent smile. "If that is your wish, it will be my delight."

He glanced at the priest. "Will you perform the ceremony, Father Joaquín?"

"It would be highly irregular, and you not even a Catholic." His pensive gaze went from Kyle to Constancia. "But...surely God would bless such a union."

Kyle went to his room to get a gold signet ring with the Renbourne crest on it. When he returned, Teresa had placed masses of garden flowers around the bed and fashioned a bouquet for her mistress. Constancia was propped up on a bank of pillows, her dark hair flowing over her shoulders. In her lace-trimmed white night robe, she looked surprisingly bridal. Her expression was rather amused, and terribly, terribly tired.

Kyle linked his fingers through Constancia's. Though he had never imagined a wedding like this one, when he looked at her haggard, lovely face, he knew this marriage was utterly right. *Till death did them part.* He choked back the thought and repeated his vows in a firm voice. The ring was enormous on her thin finger, but she closed her hand around the gold band, keeping it secure. *"Mi esposo,"* she whispered. "My husband."

He kissed her with exquisite gentleness, thinking of the years of passion and tenderness they had shared. In her eyes, he saw a mirror of those memories. His beloved, his bride. Dear God, how could he ever find such closeness again? Impossible.

The priest and servants who had acted as witnesses withdrew, leaving the newlywed couple together. Constancia closed her eyes, exhaustion etched on her face. "I can see them around me, Kyle," she said dreamily, her voice a faint thread of sound. "My parents, my sister, hovering like angels. All those I have loved and lost. So real that I wonder you cannot see them, too."

He swallowed the lump in his throat. "What matters is that you see them."

Her breathing was strained, each inhalation a visible effort. "Will you take me into the garden? I would like to see the sun and the flowers one more time."

He hesitated, thinking of the pain that had racked her for so long, but she seemed to be beyond that now. Rising, he opened the door to the courtyard, then lifted her in his arms. His bride weighed no more than a child as he carried her to the bench beneath the flowering orange tree. There he arranged her across his lap, her head on his shoulder. "Are you comfortable, Lady Maxwell?" he asked softly.

"Oh, yes." She settled against him with a sigh. The tangy sweetness of orange blossoms surrounded them. A shadow of laughter in her voice, she murmured, "Lady Maxwell. How very grand I sound."

A breeze rustled through the leaves above them, and white petals floated weightlessly down to rest on her silver-streaked hair. He kissed the top of her head, aching. She had been so much a part of his life, the epitome of feminine warmth and allure. What would he do without her? What would he regret most when she was gone?

As soon as the thought crossed his mind,

words he'd never spoken before came to his lips. "I love you, Constancia."

She tilted her head back a fraction. "I know, querido, but I didn't think you did."

Incongruously he laughed, wondering how it was possible to be simultaneously happy and devastated with grief. His laughter faded, and he realized with a sense of wonder why he'd felt that sudden passionate need to marry her—so that he could acknowledge love. "You are still entirely yourself, my dear."

"I can be no other." She paused to draw breath, then continued laboriously, "I have been so blessed, Kyle. After my family died, I thought myself cursed, driven into a life of sin and loneliness. Long after hope was gone, God sent me you, and I am whole again." She closed her eyes for a moment, then opened them again, expression burning. "I love you, my husband. And for my sake—go forth and *live!*"

"I will, mi corazón," he promised. But first, he must mourn.

She did not speak again. He held her as the shadows lengthened and petals drifted silently down, until finally he was alone.

Chapter 28

Dominic awoke, heart pounding, the scent of orange blossoms in his nostrils. It took him a moment to remember that he was at an inn near Bridgton Abbey, Lord Amworth's seat. After leaving Warfield, he'd sent Morrison back to London in the curricle with most of the baggage. The valet had gone without protest, too shaken to have any other opinions about the best course of action.

Grateful for the speed and stamina of Pegasus, Dominic had made the trip to Bridgton Abbey in less than a day. Despite his tearing anxiety to see Amworth, he forced himself to stop at a local inn for a few hours' rest and a cleanup. The situation was dire enough without him bursting in on Amworth wild-eyed and filthy.

Shaken, he sat on the edge of the bed and buried his face in his hands. Why the hell had he been dreaming of orange blossoms? Though he could not remember anything else about the dream, he still felt oppressed and miserable.

Kyle. He was feeling his brother's emotions as well as his own anxiety about Meriel. With painstaking care, he separated his churning feelings, and realized that Kyle was saturated in sorrow so intense that Dominic could taste and smell it. Yet curiously, it was not a ravaging grief. Rather, there was a sense of weary peace. Acceptance.

He closed his eyes in wordless meditation, trying to send caring and support to his brother, wherever he might be. Then he got to his feet and began to prepare for the most important meeting of his life.

Though he had decided there must be an end to deceit, for the sake of simplicity Dominic gave the footman at Bridgton Abbey one of his brother's cards. He was taken to a drawing room, where the mistress of the house joined him after a lengthy wait. Plump and pretty, Lady Amworth seemed designed by nature for smiles, but her round face showed the effects of prolonged strain.

"Lord Maxwell." She inclined her head. "I am Lady Amworth. My husband has spoken of you, of course. Have you come to inquire about his health?"

He bowed. "That, and to inform him of a situation he must know about."

She frowned. "It's about that poor girl, isn't it? I won't have my husband disturbed, Lord Maxwell. He has been deathly ill, and the outcome is still uncertain."

"Believe me, I don't want to injure his health," Dominic said fervently. "But I am sure he would want to know what I have to say."

"Very well, you may see him for a few minutes," her ladyship said grudgingly. "But if you upset him, you'll be out of Bridgton before you can blink."

Just what he needed—to be thrown out of another house. Silently he followed Lady Amworth upstairs to her husband's rooms.

Amworth was a thin, exhausted shape under the covers, but he offered a bony hand to Dominic. "You needn't look so alarmed, Maxwell," he said with dry humor. "I'm not on my deathbed yet. Elinor will not allow it." The glance he gave his wife was affectionate. "How is Meriel?"

"Sir." Dominic shook hands, then moved back a step, keeping a wary eye on Lady Amworth, who stood guard on the other side of her husband's bed. "I hope you will listen calmly, for I have no wish to move your lady wife to violence."

Amworth smiled faintly. "I shall endeavor to remain tranquil."

"First of all, I am not Kyle Renbourne, Viscount Maxwell, but Dominic Renbourne, his twin brother," Dominic said baldly. "I am deeply sorry for the deception. It was Maxwell whom you met originally, but urgent business called him away. Because of the time constraints involved in the courtship of Lady Meriel, he asked me to go to Warfield in his place."

Lady Amworth gasped, and her husband's eyes widened. "I knew that Maxwell had a younger brother, but did not know you were identical twins." His shrewd gaze went over Dominic. "That explains the vague feeling of differentness I experienced when I visited at Warfield. Was our discussion about Meriel also lies?"

"Absolutely not." Relieved that Amworth was taking news of the deception so well, Dominic continued, "My intention was to play my brother's role as quietly as possible, so that later he could return with no one the wiser. I...I didn't expect to fall in love with Meriel, but I have, and she cares for me as well.

She has opened up greatly since I arrived at Warfield—to the point where she has begun to speak."

That news was received with more shock than his announcement that he was not Kyle. Fortunately, Lady Amworth was too intrigued to evict Dominic from the sickroom. Swiftly he told them as much of what had happened as a doting uncle would approve, ending by saying, "I don't know if Meriel will marry me—she has an aversion to marriage—but she has said she will certainly not wed my brother."

Amworth frowned. "Are you seeking permission to court her in your own right?"

Dominic hesitated a moment, knowing that to answer the question would irrevocably damage his relationship with his brother. But he had no choice; Meriel must come first. "Yes, though I don't know how to convince you that I am not a fortune hunter. My inheritance is very modest compared to hers."

"It would not be a bad thing if Meriel wed a man who would live with her at Warfield," Amworth said slowly. "The one qualm I had about Maxwell was that his responsibilities would keep him in London and Dornleigh for much of the time. I might be willing to offer my blessing—if you love Meriel, and she will accept you."

"Thank you, sir," he said fervently. "I will swear any oath you wish as to the genuineness of my feelings. Meriel is...unique. Magical. I have never felt so happy, so alive...." He stopped when Amworth's amused expression showed that he was babbling.

Pulling himself back to the reason for his visit, he went on, "I came here because of a serious issue that must be resolved before there can be any more courting. Lord Grahame heard of your illness and returned to England early. When the family solicitor told him of your hopes for Meriel's marriage, he stormed up to Shropshire. Yesterday he threw me out of Warfield, and threatened my life if I ever returned."

Amworth made a rough sound that drew a frown from his wife. Holding up his hand to still her, he said, "I am in no condition to drive him out on your behalf."

Dominic smiled without humor. "I would be a poor sort of suitor if I hid behind you. Confronting Lord Grahame is my responsibility, but I felt that I would have more moral authority if I have your approval."

"My moral authority is at a low ebb now." Amworth plucked restlessly at the coverlet. "It was dishonorable to go behind Grahame's back, but I felt strongly that Meriel needed a more normal life. Though you have proved me right, Grahame is understandably angry. I doubt he'll leave Warfield simply because you ask."

Especially since Grahame considered Dominic to be Meriel's seducer, and didn't yet know that he'd been deceived as to the identity of her suitor. Dominic would deal with that when the time came. "Meriel is of age, and as mistress of Warfield she has a legal right to entertain what guests she chooses. I intend to use that fact."

"I will give you a letter authorizing you to act on my behalf where Meriel is concerned." Amworth sighed, his face strained. "Will that help?"

"It certainly will." Seeing that Lady Amworth was on the verge of ending the visit, Dominic said, "I will take my leave before I exhaust you, sir. Just one last question. Do you happen to know if General Ames is a magistrate?"

Amworth's expression eased. "He is, as well as being Grahame's former commanding officer. Perhaps you'll be able to resolve this peaceably, Renbourne."

Dominic bowed. "I hope so. It is my wish that ultimately both of Meriel's uncles will approve of her marriage. I swear that I want only the best for her."

"Wait for me downstairs," Lady Amworth said. "I shall join you shortly."

He obeyed, and was moving restlessly around the drawing room when she arrived with a folded paper in her hand. "Here is your letter. My husband dictated it to me, and signed it himself."

"Thank you, Lady Amworth." He tucked the letter in his coat. "I am very grateful to you both. I'll keep you informed."

He was on the verge of leaving when she said, "It's almost dinnertime, too late to start for Warfield. You must dine with us and spend the night."

It was an order, not a request. He smiled

wryly. "So that you can draw your own conclusions about my character?"

"Exactly so." She glanced away. "I regret that I have not been a better aunt to my husband's niece." There was a long pause before she said stiffly, "Perhaps Lady Meriel is not really mad, but...my mother was."

"You owe me no explanation, Lady Amworth," he said quietly. "Everyone has private dragons."

Her gaze returned to his face. "I begin to understand how you have drawn Meriel out. Mysterious are the ways of fate. Would Lord Maxwell have done as well with her, do you think?"

Dominic shook his head. "I doubt it. He lacks patience."

Before she could reply, the footman entered the drawing room, disapproval on his face. "A person wishes to speak to you, my lady. He says he is from Warfield Park."

Lady Amworth and Dominic exchanged puzzled glances. "Bring him in, Liddel." After the footman left, she said, "Do you suppose this could be Lord Grahame, come to castigate my husband?"

Dominic frowned. "Surely he wouldn't, knowing Lord Amworth is very ill."

She smiled humorlessly. "I doubt that would stop him. Though my husband does not complain, he has had a difficult time sharing custody of Lady Meriel with Grahame. Their opinions about her best interests were too different. There were regular clashes. Otherwise, my husband would never have arranged a marriage secretly."

Further speculation ended when the door opened and Kamal entered. With his turban and travel-stained garments, he was a startlingly foreign figure in this staid drawing room. "Kamal!" Dominic exclaimed. "Has something happened to Meriel?"

"My lady." The Indian bowed to Lady Amworth. "I came hoping to find you here, my lord, and to inform Lord Amworth that Lord Grahame has taken Lady Meriel to the asylum at Bladenham."

"My God!" Dominic froze in horror. Collecting himself, he said, "Forgive my language, Lady Amworth. Though Grahame wanted to send her to the asylum before, it didn't occur to me that he would do that when she is so much improved."

"He captured and bound her as if she were a wild beast," Kamal said, eyes glittering. "She was on her way to the asylum within an hour of your departure."

Dominic swore again, sickened by the thought of Meriel tied and caged, beating her wings against the bars until she destroyed herself. Turning to Lady Amworth, he said in a clipped voice, "I must refuse your kind hospitality, I fear. Meriel must be removed from the asylum as soon as possible."

She nodded, her face pale. "I will not tell my husband—this news might well bring on another attack, perhaps a fatal one. I rely on you to do what is necessary."

"On me, and Kamal." He glanced at the Indian. "You must be exhausted. Do you have the strength to start back tonight? There are still hours of riding time before dark."

"I shall not slow you down," Kamal said tersely.

"You two may be men of iron, but you'll need fresh horses," Lady Amworth said practically. "While they are being readied, you must both have food and drink."

She rang the bell and gave the footman orders about the horses, then ushered the men down to the kitchen. While the cook assembled a cold meal, she succinctly described the legal conditions of Meriel's guardianship. Not anticipating the massacre and Meriel's "madness," her father had taken only the standard legal precautions, meaning she was free to choose her own husband. That would simplify Dominic's task.

After Lady Amworth left them to their meal, he asked Kamal, "How did the ladies react to Grahame's actions?"

"They were most displeased with his lordship." A flash of white teeth showed in the Indian's dark beard. "Only the argument that they would hinder my journey prevented them from accompanying me."

Thank heaven that Meriel had such allies. Dominic took another slice of cold beef, then proceeded to tell Kamal who he really was.

Confession might be good for the soul, but by the time he finished enlightening everyone who had a right to know, he was going to be heartily bored with the subject.

Chapter 29

They headed straight to Bladenham, with only a short, late-night stop at a shabby inn. During the long ride, Dominic discussed strategy with Kamal. Both agreed that sheer aristocratic bluster had the best chance of success, so they descended on the asylum like a thunderstorm. As soon as the door opened, Dominic stepped inside and demanded, "I must speak to Dr. Craythorne at once."

The skinny housemaid said uncertainly, "The doctor is treating a patient, sir."

"I don't care if he's ministering to God Himself!" Dominic barked. "He will see me right now, or he'll soon be in the Shrewsbury jail."

Having modeled his behavior after Lord Wrexham at his most autocratic, Dominic wasn't surprised when the maid scuttled off in terror. It didn't hurt that Kamal was at his back, looking feral and dangerous.

Within minutes, Craythorne strode into the handsome receiving room. "What is the meaning of this intrusion?" His face changed when he saw who waited. "Lord Maxwell. I presume that you are here about Lady Meriel Grahame."

Dominic fixed the doctor with a steely glance. "You presume correctly. I want her released into my care *at once*."

"I can't do that," the doctor said calmly. "She was committed by her uncle, who is her legal guardian, and only he can authorize her release. He warned me that efforts might be made to take her away, and charged me to keep her here safely, so that she can receive the treatment she needs."

"Lord Grahame was one of Lady Meriel's guardians when she was a child, but he has no legal authority over her person now that she is of age," Dominic retorted. "Certainly he has no right to commit a healthy young woman to an asylum."

Craythorne shook his head. "You know nothing of the matter. The girl fought like a wild animal. I have seldom seen a female so demented."

"Of course she fought!" Dominic stalked forward, forcing the doctor to fall back a step. "If you were kidnapped from your home and imprisoned, wouldn't you?"

The doctor blinked, as if he hadn't thought of it that way. Recovering, he said, "Your logic is backwards. She isn't mad because she was brought here, but was brought here because she was mad. Why else would Lord Grahame commit her?"

What would persuade Craythorne? Greed was always plausible. Improvising swiftly, Dominic said, "Because Lady Meriel and I are betrothed, and Grahame wants to block our marriage. Her other uncle, Lord Amworth, approves of the match." He pulled Amworth's letter of support from his coat and gave it the doctor.

Craythorne read it twice, then handed it back,

frowning. "That's all very well, but Amworth hasn't seen her since her breakdown. He cannot know her current condition."

"Grahame's kidnapping of Meriel has nothing to do with her mental state." Letting his imagination run rampant, Dominic continued, "I believe that he has been embezzling Lady Meriel's inheritance, and he fears the audit that will take place if and when she marries. To conceal his crimes, he is trying to prevent the wedding."

After a startled moment, the doctor said, "That's absurd! A Gothic melodrama, fit only for frightening weak-minded young girls. I find it easier to believe what Grahame told me—that you are a fortune hunter determined to marry a grievously afflicted girl to gain control of her inheritance."

"The heir to Wrexham has no need to marry a fortune." Dominic's voice dropped to dangerous softness. "Would you think it Gothic for a husband to lock up his wife in a madhouse simply because she disagreed with him? Ask Jena Ames, or her father, if such a thing could happen."

Craythorne paled. "That was an unfortunate accident. The cases are quite dissimilar."

"Are they? In each case, a man brought in a woman and declared her mad, and you agreed because she tried to defend herself," Dominic said with lethal precision. "In the case of Miss Ames, I was willing to believe that you were deceived by her wicked husband, but I am no longer so sure. What kind of institution

329

are you running here, Craythorne? How many people are you holding against their will?"

"None!" the doctor replied, but he looked badly rattled. "Lady Meriel is as clearly mad as any patient I have ever seen."

"If she's mad, it's because of what you've done to her!" Dominic exploded. "I am taking her out of here right now, or as God is my witness, I will return with magistrates and militia and take this hellhole apart brick by brick! Every newspaper in Great Britain will hear the story of the distinguished physician who locks up rich women so their male relations can plunder their assets."

His voice became pure ice. "This is your last chance, Craythorne. Release Lady Meriel, or I will destroy you. The choice is yours."

The doctor looked ill. Even if he was Grahame's innocent dupe, the enmity of a powerful lord could wreck his life's work. Moistening his lips with his tongue, he said, "Come see for yourself. That will convince you of her state as no words of mine will."

"By all means, take us to her." Dominic started toward the right-hand corridor. "As I recall, females are kept in the east wing?"

"Actually, she is temporarily in the west wing." The doctor glanced at Kamal, who was following Dominic. "Your servant should wait here. Too many visitors may increase her agitation."

"Kamal is her trusted bodyguard, and her friend. His presence will be nothing but beneficial." Not to mention the fact that the

Indian would provide good support if the doctor was fool enough to use force to prevent Meriel from being taken from the asylum.

Craythorne led the way down the western hall to the heavy, metal-bound door. Dominic wanted to jump out of his skin with impatience as the doctor fumbled through his keys to find the right one.

They entered the secure area. Dominic's blood chilled as he remembered what he had seen and heard on his earlier visit. Meriel had been here for less than three days—but how long would it take for a sensitive mind to snap? How much time until a girl who had lived with near-total freedom died of captivity?

The doctor stopped in front of a door and began searching for the right key. Dominic's stomach knotted. Surely this wasn't the restraint room....

Craythorne cautioned, "Remember, this was necessary for her own safety."

The door opened to reveal Meriel's frail form tied to the chair in the center of the room. She wore a straitjacket, with additional bonds securing her to the bolted-down chair. Her face was smudged and bruised, and she stared blindly ahead, not moving a muscle when the three men entered.

"You *bastard*!" Dominic shoved past the doctor and went to her. She was like a statue, only a thready pulse in her throat showing that she was alive. Gentling his voice, he said, "We're taking you out of here, Meriel."

"She had to be restrained," Craythorne

said in a rush of nervous words. "Grahame brought her here tied in a blanket. When she was released, it took two grown men to hold her down. Without restraints, she could have injured herself badly. Besides, it's necessary to establish discipline before treatment can begin."

"Is that why her face is bruised?" Dominic said savagely as he moved behind the chair. He tried to untie the ropes, but his fingers trembled too much to manage the knot.

"Allow me, milord." A glittering dagger appeared in Kamal's hand as he joined Dominic. Craythorne gasped as the Indian began slashing through Meriel's bonds.

Dominic recognized the dagger from the time Kamal had trimmed a pineapple. Very convenient on this occasion. Not only did the razor-sharp edge make short work of the ropes, but it finished the job of cowing the doctor.

Meriel slumped forward when the last rope was cut. As Dominic knelt in front of the chair to steady her, he saw that her pupils were dilated so widely that her eyes looked black. There were stains on the straitjacket, and he thought he detected the sweetish odor of laudanum. "Did you force one of your damned narcotic potions down her?"

"I was just trying to calm her enough to begin treatment," the doctor said defensively. "You have no idea how difficult it is to work with mad patients."

"And if they aren't mad to begin with, they will be by the time you're done with them,"

Dominic growled as Kamal sliced through the straitjacket that immobilized her arms. Together they peeled the damnable thing off Meriel.

She tumbled forward onto Dominic, locking her arms around his neck and her legs around his waist. Her slim body was shaking as if from fever.

He crushed her close, desperately grateful that she was safe. She seemed unbearably fragile as she buried her face in the angle between his neck and shoulder. What if this captivity had destroyed all the progress she had made? What if the girl he'd fallen in love with was gone beyond recall?

Unable to bear the thought, he whispered huskily, "Just a little longer, sprite. Then you'll be out of this foul place forever."

It was awkward rising from a crouch with her clinging like a monkey, but he managed. "If you've caused permanent harm, Craythorne..." He let the implied threat dangle menacingly in the air.

"I'll admit that she seems to recognize you," the doctor said grudgingly. "If any of my people had released her from the restraints, she'd have attacked like a wolverine. But that doesn't mean she's sane."

"Could *you* prove you were sane, Craythorne? I doubt it," Dominic said caustically. "How long until the narcotic wears off?"

Craythorne hesitated. "Several hours at least. The dosage was heavy for someone so small."

Without another glance in the doctor's direction, Dominic left the restraint room, Kamal close behind. Craythorne made no attempt to stop them as they left the building. He was probably as anxious to be rid of his unwelcome guests as they were eager to go.

Kamal brought the horses, and Dominic found that it really wasn't possible to mount with a female holding on to him. He passed her to Kamal and got on his horse, then took her in his arms again. It would be awkward to have her across his lap, but he couldn't let her ride pillion when she was drugged.

Dominic and Kamal didn't speak until they had left the asylum property and were on the public road. Then Kamal said, "The doctor will send word to Lord Grahame immediately."

"I know." Dominic glanced down at the top of Meriel's flaxen head and wondered how long it would be until she could bear to look anyone in the eye again. If she weren't so weak, they could have gone to Warfield, but he couldn't do that with her in this condition. Where to go instead? Certainly not a public inn—it would be too easy for Grahame to find them. He forced his weary brain to think. "We'll take her to Holliwell Grange. It's not far, and the general will help us, I believe."

Kamal nodded agreement, and they set off. A good thing the grange was near, because the horses were too tired to go far or fast. Dominic tried not to think about his own exhaustion. There would be time enough for that when Meriel was safe.

The Ameses reacted to their unexpected visitors with the swift common sense of a military family. After hearing Dominic's explanation of why they had come, Jena hustled Meriel away for tending. Meriel was still close to sleepwalking, but she went willingly. Dominic took it as a good sign that she knew her friends from her enemies.

Though he was reeling with fatigue after the long journey to and from Bridgton Abbey, Dominic couldn't rest until the truth was known. "There is something else you must know, General." Tersely he explained who he was.

After a startled moment, Ames said, "You don't believe in a simple life, do you? We can talk about this in the morning. Right now, you both need to rest."

Grateful to accept the general's judgment, Dominic followed him to a bedroom. Within two minutes, he washed, stripped, and was sleeping like the dead.

Chapter 30

Flames and screams and a silhouette of evil. Traveling in terror through the desert night, a large hand on her spine to prevent her falling from the saddlebow of a horse so rough-gaited she could barely breathe. Crying for her mama and papa, and a frantic refusal to believe they would never come. Hope eroding day by day, until there was nothing left but bitter acceptance that she had been abandoned.

The scene shifted to her uncle lashing ropes around her blanket-wrapped body. Fighting frantically to escape before the horrible straitjacket, but being overpowered. The doctor speaking soothingly as he rammed a funnel down her throat and poured a sticky potion that she must swallow or die of choking.

This time, she knew better than to expect rescue.

She returned to consciousness in broken patches, cold with sweat. But this time, rescue *had* come, hadn't it? Or had she imagined Renbourne's embrace, his scent, and the steady beat of his heart under her ear?

Eyes closed, she took stock. A soft bed, a small dark room with a dim light. A clean country smell rather than the stone-deep despair of the asylum. Warily she opened her eyes and saw Jena Ames sitting by her bed, quietly reading by the light of an oil lamp. So Renbourne and Kamal really had come for her.

She tried to order her chaotic thoughts. Kamal had brandished a lethal dagger, and a furious Renbourne had been on the verge of ripping out the doctor's throat. Another ride on horseback, but this time cradled against Renbourne instead of weeping helplessly on a terrifying ride into the unknown.

Then Jena, who helped her wash and made her drink broth before tucking her into bed. She shifted her gaze and saw that she wore an overlarge shift, old but clean.

Cautiously she stretched. All her muscles ached from the torment of being tied like a mummy for hours. The only respite had been periodic releases from the chair when a burly female attendant had helped her use a chamber pot, a clumsy, humiliating business for someone tied in a straitjacket.

Hearing Meriel's movement, Jena glanced up. "You're awake. Good." She bent forward to study Meriel's eyes. "It looks as if most of the laudanum has worn off. How do you feel?"

Meriel gave an infinitesimal shrug.

"You're probably thirsty." Jena poured a glass of water, then held it to Meriel's lips. "My mouth was always horribly dry after they made me take one of those ghastly potions." Though she tried to speak calmly, there was a faint tremor in her voice. It hadn't been that long since she had been as helpless as Meriel.

As Meriel greedily swallowed the water, she tried to remember how long Jena had been in the asylum. Many months. Meriel had been there—two days? three?—and had already vanished into the mists of her own mind. She would never have survived a year.

After Meriel drank her fill, Jena set the glass aside. "I was horrified when Renbourne and Kamal appeared. You looked more dead than alive. How *dare* your uncle send you to Bladenham! You and I both owe your young man a great deal."

So they knew who he really was. Good. Meriel thought of Renbourne with sharp longing. His physical presence had lured her from the seductive blankness of the mists. Reassured her that this time she had not been abandoned to her fate.

Where was he now?

"Knowing you were in the asylum has brought it all back." Jena gazed at the lamp, her expression strained. "I've been trying to...to come to terms with my time there. Dr. Craythorne isn't evil—in his own way, I think he's compassionate and very dedicated. Many of the patients really were hopelessly mad, but he is so single-minded that he sees madness everywhere, even when it doesn't exist. That I can't forgive."

She looked at Meriel again, forcing a smile. "I shouldn't talk of that. More amusing to tell you how we're going to turn the tables on my ghastly husband. Since divorce is virtually impossible, my father's solicitor has filed to get me an annulment. Did you know a marriage isn't legal if one of the parties is insane at the time of the wedding? Since my own husband committed me to an asylum, I must have been mad. Ergo, the marriage was invalid." She smiled wryly. "I had no trouble signing an affidavit that I was insane when I married—I had to have been crazy to marry Morton."

Meriel smiled a little, understanding Jena's amusement. There was poetic justice to the grounds used for the petition for annulment. She hoped it was granted. How horrible to be forever tied to a man one loathed.

Jena studied her face. "One of the things I hated most about Bladenham was the lack of privacy. Knowing that at any time an attendant might peer through the window in the door to see what I was doing. I didn't want you to wake up alone, but now that the drug has worn off, would you rather I left you?"

Meriel gave a sharp nod.

"You're almost yourself again. In fact, we're having a real conversation." Jena hesitated, then said diffidently, "Mr. Renbourne said that you're speaking now. I don't suppose you'd like to demonstrate?"

Meriel shifted her gaze to the faded wallpaper. She wasn't prepared to talk to anyone other than Renbourne.

Correctly interpreting her silence, Jena got to her feet. "Perhaps another time. Try to get more rest. By morning, the last of the potion should have worn off." She leaned forward and kissed Meriel's cheek. "I'm in the room on your left, Mr. Renbourne is across the hall, and my father and Kamal are in the other wing, so you're safe. No one can kidnap you from Holliwell Grange. If you need anything, just call."

She started to lift the lamp, then hesitated. "Shall I leave the light?"

Meriel nodded again. She'd had enough of shadows.

After Jena left, she lay still for a time, appreciating the silence and cleanliness and privacy—and giving Jena time to undress and go to bed.

The knowledge that Renbourne was across the hall made her...hungry. She wanted him. Wanted his touch, his taste, his closeness.

When she thought enough time had passed, she shakily sat up and swung her legs over the side of the bed. Though her body hurt as if it had been pounded from head to foot, she felt a certain detachment from the pain. A lingering effect of the drug, perhaps.

Cautiously she stood, and had to grab the bedside table to keep from falling. When her balance steadied, she made her way to the washstand and splashed water on her face. The coolness helped clear her head.

As she dried her hands and face, she studied herself in the small mirror above the washstand. She looked ghostly in the dim light. Her only color was a purple bruise on one cheekbone and dark shadows beneath her eyes. With tendrils of hair escaping from her braid to writhe around her face, she was a sight to make Mrs. Marks sigh with exasperation. But seeing the image made her feel real. Returned from the mists.

Cautiously she opened the door. No squeaks. She stepped across the hall and turned the knob on the opposite door. It swung open soundlessly; the general's household was as well run as his army cantonment must have been.

She closed the door and leaned against it as her eyes adjusted to the darker room. Renbourne lay sprawled on his side on the bed, illuminated by a wash of moonlight. The blanket had worked its way down to his waist, exposing his bare torso. Judging by the pile of crumpled garments, he had simply stripped off his clothing and fallen into bed.

She liked the way he was made, broad through the shoulders, narrow through the hips. The clean limbs and firm muscles of a man who enjoyed physical work. In the moonlight the fading patterns of the mehndi on his upper chest were faintly visible, a reminder of the intimacy they had shared.

Being in the same room, breathing the same air, brought a sharp release of tension. When her uncle drove Renbourne from Warfield, she'd been terrified that he was leaving forever. Certainly she hadn't expected him to discover what had happened to her, and come to the rescue. The thought made her soften with tenderness.

Craving the feel of his bare skin against hers, she peeled off the loose shift and climbed into the bed. Trying not to disturb him, she carefully fitted her body against his, circling his ribs with one arm so that her breasts pressed into his back, tucking her knee between his thighs. Then she relaxed, finally feeling safe. His scent, warm and familiar, created a hazy feeling of contentment.

Dreamily she stroked his chest, enjoying the contrast of smooth warm skin and soft, springy hair. Despite her relaxation, she felt paradoxically alive.

She kissed the hollow under his shoulder blade, savoring the salty taste of his skin. What had begun as a desire for simple closeness became more as her blood quickened. Could a male mate in his sleep? It would be an amusing experiment to find out.

She skimmed the firm shape of his flank under the blanket, then moved her hand up the front of his thigh until she found what she sought. Already semi-erect, his organ hardened in her hand. The memory of their previous mating sprang to vivid life as she began to caress him. She wanted—*needed*—that intimate fire again.

"Meriel," Renbourne murmured. Rolling onto his back, he drew her close and began to caress one breast with his other hand.

He wasn't truly awake, but his instincts were excellent. She raised her head and kissed him. His lips, warm and welcoming, aroused her. She wanted to flow in and around him, dissolve all barriers until they were truly one flesh.

His hand glided over her belly and came to rest between her legs, producing a rush of liquid heat. As his fingers slid deep inside her, she sucked in her breath, stunned at the swiftness of her response. No longer playing, she nipped his earlobe.

He came awake with a jolt. "My God, you're really here!" he breathed. "I thought I was dreaming." He kissed her with dark velvet richness.

Exhilaration blazed through her. Yes, *yes!* She wanted to eat him alive, ravish him until Bladenham was seared from her mind. She rolled on top of him, her legs bracketing his...

And learned that his damned conscience had woken up, too. He caught her shoulders, fingers tight. In a low voice laced with laughter and desire, he said, "I assume this means you've recovered."

She shivered with delight. Teasing him when he was asleep was all very well, but so much better to have him fully present, concentrated on her. She kissed his throat, enjoying the whiskery rasp of his unshaved chin. So *male*. Delicious.

He lifted her so that their upper bodies no longer touched, and caught her gaze. "We mustn't do this," he said firmly. "I swore I wouldn't compromise you again. Marriage or nothing, sprite. Besides, this seems like an abuse of General Ames's hospitality. He would not like knowing I took advantage of you under his roof."

Did being a gentleman mean he always thought it was his fault if they mated? She snorted at the absurdity of that and ground her hips into his so that her lushly lubricated female parts slid along the silky length of his erection. The mind-melting intimacy made her whimper with pleasure, and gave her a fierce craving for more.

He went rigid, and she felt a hot throb where their organs touched. So close, yet not close enough. She wriggled, frantically trying to take him inside her. Then his hands locked hard on her hips, preventing further motion.

"Stop that, you little witch," he said hoarsely. "This is not right."

The moonlight revealed a face of tight, sweat-slicked planes as he struggled to control his body. How strong he was, to be able to wrestle passion, and win. She didn't have a tithe of his discipline.

She felt his muscles tighten as he started to remove her, and felt as if he were ripping her in half, tearing her away from her most vital self. "Please," she whispered, humiliated at how desperately she needed him. "Please, Dominic."

As he hesitated, hot silent tears spilled from her eyes and fell onto his chest. Pain spasmed across his face. Then he drew her down so that her breasts crushed against him. "Don't cry, sweeting," he said unsteadily. "Please don't cry."

Dizzy with relief, she kissed him with devouring intensity. Was it love, that he could resist passion but not her desperate plea? There was so much to learn from him, so much. More than she could master in a lifetime.

Hand trembling with impatience, she guided him inside her. A moan of astonished delight escaped her as she slowly lowered herself onto his shaft. Her body accommodated him more easily this time, clasping with seductive heat. She moved her hips experimentally. He groaned as she slid up and down with sensual ease, taking him as deep as she could. She liked the sense of power, the fantasy that she could enslave him with pleasure, as he had done for her.

His eyes closed, but he cupped her breasts, caressing with strong, clever fingers that sent frissons of excitement scorching through her veins until they fused with the fire in her loins. And there was something special about this position, this angle, the way their bodies rubbed together...

The illusion of power vanished as her body escaped her control. Every ounce of her was moving, writhing, pulsing in a divine dance where he was the only imaginable partner, a mate who enriched and humbled her.

Faster...

Harder...

Splintering...

Falling...but not alone. Ah, God, *not alone.*

He held her to him, shaking. He had not known that passion could be so...so shattering. Some of that intensity came from the fear he had experienced on her behalf, and his profound gratitude at having her safe again. But mostly it was Meriel herself.

He'd never known a woman who was so totally absorbed when she made love. She had no self-consciousness, no calculation about who was winning the silent battle that often lurked beneath the surface when men and women came together. She gave herself to him utterly—and there was no greater aphrodisiac.

He liked having her rest on top of him—she was just a little bit of a thing, albeit all woman—but her skin was beginning to feel chilled in the breeze from the open window. Rolling to his side, he folded her against him spoon style and pulled the blanket over them both. She gave a throaty sigh and snuggled back into the curve of his body.

Marveling at how well she had survived her ordeal, he kissed her temple. "No permanent damage sustained at the asylum?"

After a lengthy silence, she said, "Not damage, but...change. Because I have had such freedom for so long, I didn't know how...how vulnerable I was. It only took one damnable man to wrench me out of paradise."

His arm tightened around her. "They say the road to hell is paved with good intentions, and it's certainly true here. Your uncle's good intentions sent you to hell."

She shivered. "I want to go home."

He sighed, knowing that she wasn't going to like what he had to say. "That won't be easy, sprite. After leaving Warfield I visited Lord Amworth and enlisted his support on your behalf. I intended to return and ask General Ames to join me in his capacity as magistrate while I politely explained to Lord Grahame that you are sane, of legal age, and entitled to have any guests you choose."

Her head nodded vigorously.

He smiled ruefully. "It's no longer that simple. Kamal found me at Bridgton Abbey and told me you'd been sent to the asylum. Dr. Craythorne is a well-known specialist in mental disorders, and he thinks you're mad. With Craythorne's opinion as evidence, Lord

Grahame could go to a different magistrate and argue that I abducted you from the asylum in order to seize control over your property. I'm no expert on the law, but if there is a dispute, you might be made a ward of the Crown until it's settled." He took a deep breath. "You might be returned to an asylum."

She went rigid in his arms. *"No!"*

He hated frightening her with the possibilities, but she had to be made to understand. "Legal disputes are not settled quickly, Meriel. Though Amworth would try to help, his health is still very fragile. Grahame might get his way through sheer bullheadedness. His opinion of me will become even lower when he learns that I'm not Lord Maxwell. Most of the world will agree with him."

"No," she said again, but this time her voice was a whisper. "You won't let them put me in the madhouse again, would you?"

"I can only think of two ways to save you from that, Meriel," he said soberly. "The first is to take you away, and live in hiding." They'd be in very modest circumstances, too, given the state of his finances, but he didn't mention that.

She made a hissing sound. "I won't be driven from Warfield!"

He'd known she would feel that way. "Which means there is really only one choice." He took a deep breath. "You'll have to marry me."

Her heart accelerated under his hand. "I do not wish to marry."

"I know, but marriage is the only way I have any standing to help you, Meriel," he

347

explained. "As the seducer of an innocent, I'm a villain. As your husband, I have not only the right, but the responsibility, to protect you."

She slid from his embrace and climbed from the bed, going to stand by the window. In the moonlight, she was a slim silvery shadow. He winced at the dark bruises that marred the perfection of her pale body. She had fought her kidnappers with the fierceness of her warrior ancestors.

After a long silence, she asked quietly, "Is my danger so great, or do you exaggerate to force me to marry?"

After a hard look at his conscience, he replied, "The danger is real, Meriel. I wish it weren't, because duress is a poor way to start a marriage."

He got out of bed and joined her at the window, resting his hands on her shoulders as he gazed over her head. "I'd much rather persuade you with sweet reason and sweeter kisses, and I'm arrogant enough to think that in time you would decide becoming a wife would not be so very bad." He kissed her lightly on the temple.

She sighed. "I would prefer to be your mistress."

He smiled wryly, glad that neither of her chaperons was around to hear such a shocking comment. "That isn't one of the available choices, Meriel. Your uncle may already be searching for you, possibly with a warrant for my arrest."

Shivering, she crossed her arms on her

chest. "So I must choose between the devil I know and the devil I don't know."

He wondered which of those was him. "I will sign a marriage settlement that leaves control of your property with you and your trustees so that I can't plunder your inheritance, if that's what you fear."

"You offered that once before," she said without inflection.

Her tone made him realize that even more than wealth, she cherished the freedom of her old life. Recognizing what must be done, he said, "I give you my solemn word that if you ever decide you don't want me at Warfield, you have only to ask me to leave, and I will go. I will not claim any rights over either your fortune or your body."

She lifted her head and gazed at the moon, her expression cool and remote. "So you are willing to become my defender, and demand nothing of me in return?"

"Yes." Even though some future whim of hers could leave him alone, not free to seek another wife because he was bound to a woman who no longer wanted him. It was a bleak prospect, yet he could not abandon her to her uncle's relentless sense of duty.

She swallowed, throat flexing like a silver column in the moonlight. "Very well, Dominic. I will marry you."

It was what he had wanted desperately. Why, then, did her acceptance leave him aching with sadness?

Chapter 31

Meriel awoke the next morning in her original bed. Renbourne must have carried her back after she fell asleep. So very conventional. But perhaps he was right. She'd lived an unconventional life for years, and now she was paying the price.

Worse, Renbourne might also pay a heavy price. She had not realized, until he mentioned the topic in passing, that he might be in serious trouble for aiding her. Lord Grahame had been furious with him—very likely he would try to have Renbourne arrested for "kidnapping" an heiress. Or worse. She had a swift, horrific image of a duel, and Renbourne's body bleeding on the ground.

No.

She climbed from the bed, expression set. She had drawn Renbourne into danger, and now she must do whatever was necessary to resolve the situation. Her days as a wild child of nature, who understood more than anyone realized, were over. For better or worse, she was now part of the wider world. The sooner she learned its ways, the better for everyone who had generously come to her aid.

Her own garments had been ruined by her stay in the asylum, so Jena had borrowed clothing from a housemaid. After washing up, Meriel donned the coarse shift and faded blue dress without enthusiasm. The garments hung on her, for even the smallest Holliwell

Grange maid was obviously much more robust than she.

Worse than the dress were crude stockings and slippers. With a sigh, she put them on, for soon she would be going places where bare feet would not be practical. The footwear would have been welcome in Bladenham, for the flagstone floors had been wretchedly cold, especially for someone who couldn't warm herself by movement.

Jena had also provided a brush and comb, so Meriel put her hair in order. Then, as respectable as she could manage, she went downstairs to join the world of normal people.

Renbourne and the Ameses were in the dining room eating breakfast, and Kamal also. Though he was respected at Warfield, he was still considered a servant. At Holliwell, a less grand establishment, he was being treated as an honored guest. Perhaps that was because Jena and the general had lived in India and saw him differently.

When she entered the dining room door, everyone turned to look at her. She stopped, flushing, and remembered why she had chosen to avoid society. Then Jena rose from the table with a smile. "It's hard to believe how much improved you look, Meriel. You're just in time to join the war council."

A good thing she had come down, since it was her life being discussed. After choosing a soft-boiled egg and a hot muffin from the sideboard, Meriel took the cup of tea Jena poured and sat down opposite Renbourne.

He smiled at her with intimate warmth. "I've just finished the whole story of how we came to show up on the Ames's doorstep last night." He watched her carefully. "I also told them that we've decided to marry."

Ames frowned. "That's the best solution, but is it your wish, Lady Meriel?"

The general wasn't sure whether or not she was mentally competent, she realized. It was time to jump another fence. She swallowed hard. "Yes."

"So you *can* talk!" Jena said with delight. "We must have a good gossip soon. I can chatter for two, but it will be more fun if you answer."

Meriel glanced at Kamal and saw amusement in his dark eyes. He was not surprised that she was capable of speech. Had he always known how much of her apparent witlessness was from choice? Probably, yet he had let her be as she wished. One could not ask for a better friend.

Renbourne looked relieved, as if he'd been half expecting her to change her mind. Breaking open a muffin, he said, "Obviously the sooner we marry, the better. The question is where. We could go to London and get a special license, or travel to Scotland, where we can be married without waiting. From here, Scotland isn't much farther than London, so I think that's the best choice."

Jena shook her head doubtfully. "A Gretna Green marriage carries a stigma that you'll never live down."

"It would also reinforce the appearance

that you're a fortune hunter, and Lady Meriel is a helpless victim," the general added. "London would be better."

Dominic hesitated. "London is a dirty, smelly, noisy place at the best of times. It will seem far worse to someone who has lived for many years in the country."

Heads turned to Meriel, and there was a murmur of agreement. They all thought she was incapable of surviving the rigors of the city.

Before Meriel could offer her own opinion, the general raised one hand. "No more discussion. You may borrow my carriage, but I don't want to know which destination you choose. As a magistrate, I must tell the truth if Grahame comes and asks me if I know where the pair of you are. Better not to know."

"It's very good of you to help us, General Ames," Renbourne said soberly.

"You saved Jena. I will not see another girl locked wrongly in a madhouse." The general's eagle gaze went to Meriel. "But my aid is conditional on further speech with Lady Meriel. When you've finished eating, my dear, walk with me in the garden."

It was an order, not a suggestion. Meriel's muffin suddenly tasted like sawdust. Now that she had officially become a rational being, people wanted to *talk* to her. Mostly they wanted to tell her what to do. But there was no retreating now. Washing the last of her muffin down with tea, she said, "Very well."

She gave Renbourne a darkling glance, intending to convey that she did not wish him to completely rearrange her life in her absence, then went outside with General Ames. She remembered him from her family's visit to Cambay, and even then he'd made her nervous. Like her uncle Grahame, he had a steely energy that made her want to fade quietly into the shrubbery.

Perhaps sensing her nerves, at first he strolled in silence, a silver-headed cane in one hand. Though the garden was only a few acres, it was well laid out and carefully tended, with winding paths designed to make the area appear larger than it was. Even the kitchen garden pleased the eye, with neat beds and plump produce.

The path came to a stone wall espaliered with fruit trees. The general stopped and studied the ripening peaches on the first espalier. "When you came to Cambay with your parents, you were an intrepid child on a white pony. More than a year later, you returned looking like a waxen doll. Though I hoped you would recover in time, when I retired here to Holliwell the county was rife with stories of the mad Lady Meriel." He looked at her askance. "Now you are a young lady on the verge of marriage. How do all those different Meriels go together?"

She frowned, unsure how to answer. "All are me."

"Do you remember the attack at Alwari?"

She gave him a narrow-eyed glance. "Why?"

His jaw tightened. "I've never forgiven myself for the fact that your parents died so

354

close to Cambay. Only a day's travel away. They should have been safe so near a major British cantonment, but they weren't. As commanding officer, I felt responsible."

Did men always feel responsible for everything? Apparently. She thought, chilled, of gunshots and flames and screaming. "The raiders knew exactly what they did. They would not have been easily stopped."

Ames ground his cane into the turf. "We investigated, of course. Apparently the attackers were bandits unofficially sanctioned by the princely state of Kanphar. The Maharajah of Kanphar allowed the bandits refuge in his hill country. In return, they didn't attack his people, and he received part of their loot. Naturally the maharajah denied that—butter wouldn't have melted in his mouth—but it's devilish odd that you turned up in Kanphar's palace. He claimed you were a gift from another ruler, and that he sent you to Cambay as soon as he realized you were English. Was that true?"

She shook her head. "I was taken directly to the Kanphar zenana."

Ames scowled. "I wanted to march in and annex the blasted place, but we had no proof, and there were political reasons for accepting Kanphar's explanations." He stabbed the cane into the turf again. "A pack of damned lies. I had to order your uncle Grahame to stay away from Kanphar. He'd acted as liaison to the maharajah's court, but after your parents died, he wanted to go in and torch the palace. A good thing he had to return to England to take up his duties, or he might have started a war."

An elusive thought shimmered in Meriel's mind like a silver fish, then disappeared. When she tried to recapture it, she came up with a faint memory of her two uncles taking custody of her at a London hotel. She'd barely been aware of them, preferring to play with the flowers Kamal had bought for her. After months on shipboard, she had yearned for the scent and feel of greenery.

The general began to walk along the path that paralleled the stone wall. "You're sure you want to marry young Renbourne?"

She had said so earlier, hadn't she? Not only did people want to talk—they asked the same questions over and over. "You think him unworthy?"

"I've commanded a great many young men in my time, and I can tell when one is sound." The general picked a daisy from a vibrant clump. "Renbourne has character and honor, and he obviously loves you. But while his birth is respectable, his fortune is vastly inferior to yours. Does that bother you?"

"Why can a rich man marry a poor woman with little comment, but not the reverse?" she asked dryly.

"Good point. Maybe because rich young orphan girls seem in need of protection." With a hint of smile, he presented her with the daisy. "Or because a young girl's sweet self is considered dowry enough."

She sniffed, thinking it more likely that society considered it natural law for a man to support his wife, and was uncomfortable when that was reversed. Such nonsense. "Why do you question the match?"

"Renbourne will take care of you well." Ames coughed uncomfortably. "But this is very sudden. You've had a sheltered life. In marriage...well, a wife has duties. You're very young...."

She blinked, astonished. "You doubt I can perform my wifely duties?"

The general's leathery face colored. "You don't have a mother, after all. Perhaps Jena should talk to you."

Meriel wanted to burst into laughter. So this fierce old general was concerned with her virgin innocence. She was tempted to say that she had already found "marital duties" much to her liking, and it was Renbourne who had needed protection from her, not the reverse. Though the previous night, after she had accepted his proposal, he had carried her back to his bed and demonstrated exactly how masterful he could be when his conscience was no longer chiding him....

Giving herself a mental shake, she said gravely, "I am not so young as I appear, General Ames, and have lived much with nature."

Eager to relinquish the topic, he nodded brusquely. "As long as you understand what you are getting into."

They reached a fork in the path. When the general turned left, on the branch that curved back to the house, Meriel said, "I wish to walk more."

He hesitated. "Don't go too far. I expect that Renbourne will want to be off very soon. I need to order the arrangements."

Without even a semblance of good-bye, she headed down the right-hand path. Rather desperately, she needed to be alone.

Chapter 32

Meriel followed the flagstone path on a rambling route that led through lush banks of flowers. Just beyond a pleasantly shaded wooden bench, the path ended in a circular area defined by high box hedges. Inside were borders of roses, and a gently weathered stone fountain of a small boy holding a dolphin.

With a sigh, she flopped onto the grass that surrounded the fountain. Less than an hour of being normal, and already she had tired of it. Defiantly she pulled off slippers and stockings so that she could feel the cool, living grass under her feet. Ahhh, heaven.

She lay back full length on the soft turf and idly watched a pair of small white butterflies dancing around each other in mad abandon, flying higher and higher until they soared far above the hedges. Nature was in a mating frame of mind.

The gentle plash of water from the dolphin's mouth into the pool below eased the tension that had been building inside her. She must become stronger, or the demands of the world would overwhelm her. Was normality worth it?

Perhaps not...but Renbourne was. Memory of the tenderness and passion between them the night before made her shiver despite the warm sun. Being with him felt so *right*. Though she had lived with little or no human closeness for most of her life, now that she had experienced it, she didn't want to let it go. A pity that he and she couldn't be together without marriage, but from the way everyone acted, she was resigned to the fact that he must be right about that.

She was reluctantly thinking about returning to the house when she heard the sound of voices. A man and woman, coming toward her. As the voices became clearer, she recognized Jena and Kamal. She sat up on the grass and frowned at her footwear. No, she'd stay barefoot for a while.

Jena's voice said, "It's a lovely morning. Let's sit on the bench for a while."

Meriel heard the creak of wood as two bodies settled on the bench just outside the fountain garden. She peered through a small gap in the hedge. The bench was less than ten feet away, so she could see Jena and Kamal clearly. Though the two were at opposite ends of the bench, she sensed an interesting awareness between them.

If she were a real lady, she would announce her presence. Not yet being a lady, she toyed with the daisy the general had given her, hoping they would go away.

Jena tilted her face up, absorbing the sun's rays. "After being in the asylum, I take nothing for granted. Everything seems precious. Fresh air. Sunshine. The freedom to come and go as I please."

"You would not have liked an Indian zenana," Kamal said in his deep voice. "For women who lived in one, there was sunshine and comfort, but little freedom."

"I have visited women in zenanas. I would go mad in such a place." After a silence, Jena turned her head to Kamal. "From our discussions, it is clear that you are an educated man. Surely you could have achieved high rank in your own country. Why were you willing to leave your home for a distant land?"

Kamal hesitated, as if wondering how to answer. "I *had* achieved high rank, and it meant a life of war. Then I took Lady Meriel to Cambay, and was asked if I would escort her and her chaperon back to England. I realized fate was offering me a chance to live a life of peace." So softly the words were almost inaudible, he added, "And penance."

Meriel studied his calm profile, fascinated. How could she not have known this about him? But she had never thought to ask questions, for Kamal had been so much a part of her life. She would as soon have questioned the rain or the wind.

Jena asked, "Do you ever regret coming to England?"

He smiled. "There is nothing more peaceful than a garden. I chose the right path."

"I'm glad." Jena paused, then said, "Did you know my mother was Hindu? I am as much Indian as English."

"I had wondered." Kamal studied her face. "Jena is a Hindu name, and your heritage is suggested in your coloring and your features."

"I think my mixed blood was part of the reason my husband treated me so badly," she said brittlely. "Morton didn't know I was half-Indian when we married. Not that I lied—it just didn't seem important. After he learned the truth, it was as if...as if he considered me no longer fully human. And not only was I a mongrel, but I defied him! Easy to condemn such a wife to a madhouse."

"I'm sorry," Kamal said quietly. "The world is too often a cruel place."

Jena brushed back her dark hair with fingers that weren't quite steady. "I'm not sorry now that I am free. I am rid of Morton, and will not make such a mistake again."

"One is stronger for mistakes."

She laughed. "Then I should be capable of lifting mountains!"

"I would think you capable of almost anything."

Their gazes locked. A pulse visible in her throat, Jena asked haltingly, "Forgive me this impertinence, Kamal, but it has been said that you are a eunuch. Yet from what little I know, you do not...not have the appearance."

No woman would ask such a question

without a powerful reason. Meriel held her breath as she watched, feeling intense emotions swirling around the couple on the bench.

Unexpectedly, Kamal grinned. "My little lady's chaperon, a Mrs. Madison, took it into her head that I was a guard from the zenana. Thinking a eunuch would be considered a more fit guardian for a little girl, I never corrected her error."

Jena gave a peal of laughter. "How wicked of you! Yet it worked, for I think you were Meriel's salvation."

"I hope so. She is as dear to me as a child of my body."

The implications of getting and bearing a child stilled the air between them, and there was a taut silence as Jena and Kamal regarded each other. Then, with painful uncertainty, she touched his large brown hand where it lay on the bench between them. The gesture was light, and could easily be ignored if he chose.

Instead, Kamal slowly turned his palm upward and clasped Jena's hand. Nothing more. Yet there was unmistakable tenderness and promise in his response.

Light flared between them, joining their energies into one even though only their hands touched. Stunned, Meriel sat back on her heels and considered what she had witnessed. Jena and Kamal? To her, Kamal was a kind and infinitely patient friend, almost a father. But he was also a strong, attractive man, and not old. To Jena, half Indian herself, he was not even foreign.

Before Meriel had met Renbourne, she would have not have comprehended that unruly attraction between a man and woman. If she had witnessed the scene between Jena and Kamal, she would have been resentful and confused, for Kamal's care and kindness had always been for *her*.

But her life had changed, and she no longer needed so much from him. She had found a deeper intimacy with Renbourne. If Kamal wished for that kind of closeness with a woman, was he not entitled after all his self-less generosity?

She wrapped her arms around her knees and rocked, wondering what kind of future the pair might have if they desired greater closeness. As long as Jena had a husband, there could be no formal relationship, but Renbourne had said that women of experience could have irregular connections as long as they were discreet.

If Jena's marriage was annulled—and from what Meriel had seen of General Ames, it was likely that he had the will and the connections to ensure that happened—Jena would be free to marry again if she wished. Though it would be unusual for an English gentlewoman to marry an Indian, her father could hardly object, since he'd done the same. How very exotic for staid Shropshire!

A truly worldly thought occurred to Meriel. If she became a "normal" member of society, the wealthy daughter of an earl with an equally well-born husband, she would have social power in the county. If she wished to extend her friendship to an uncommon couple—a general's daughter and her foreign husband—most, perhaps all, of the local gentry would follow. With wry amusement, she recognized that if one was part of society, it was best to belong to the upper echelons and have power to help one's friends.

With a click like a key fitting into a lock, she suddenly understood why Renbourne wanted her as wife, not mistress. To be husband and wife was a declaration to the world, a statement that they belonged together. He had said as much, but she hadn't truly grasped what he meant. Though Meriel didn't share his respect for marriage—look how badly Jena's husband had behaved—she better understood his point of view.

Her thoughts were interrupted when she heard Kamal say, "It is time we found milady and took her back to the house."

"I wonder where she can be—it's not so large a garden that she could go far." Jena caught her breath. "Heavens, you don't think she's back by the fountain, do you?"

"There is but one way to find out." The bench creaked as weight came off it.

Meriel's heart jumped with alarm. Even good friends would not like the fact that she had eavesdropped on such private moments. But there was nowhere to run—the fountain circle was in the corner of the larger garden and had only one entrance.

Barely in time, she took the only course

possible and curled up on her side in the grass as if she'd fallen asleep in the sun, the daisy in one hand. With effort she made her breathing even, keeping her eyes closed as footsteps approached.

Kamal said softly, "She sleeps."

"Probably still feeling the effects of the drugs from the asylum," Jena said with equal softness. "She looks tired."

They were being so kind that Meriel felt a stab of guilt at her eavesdropping. Perhaps some of the social conventions she'd scorned had legitimate uses—such as not violating the privacy of others.

"No need to wake her." Kamal's strong arms lifted her, as they had so often when she was a child. She made a small show of coming partially awake, and tucked the daisy into his beard. Then she cuddled into his shoulder as he carried her back to the house.

With sadness, she realized that he might never again carry her like this. Though he had been her rock and her refuge, both of them were moving forward into new lives, and the relationship between them would change.

Change *hurt*.

During Meriel's walk, all arrangements had been made for the journey, including a portmanteau of hastily collected garments for the future bride. There was a brief discussion on whether or not Kamal would accompany them, but he decided it was more important to return quietly to Warfield and reassure the ladies that Meriel was well. A similar message had already been sent to Lord and Lady Amworth.

Well before midmorning, the carriage rumbled down the drive of Holliwell Grange, and they were on their way. Meriel had donned stockings and shoes again in honor of the leave-taking, but even before they reached the main road, she'd pulled them off and was wriggling her toes in relief.

Renbourne smiled and took her hand. "You must be frayed to the bone with so much socializing and shoe wearing."

She nodded, glad that he understood. Except for Kamal, he was the only person whose company didn't tire her. In fact, when Renbourne was near, she felt...energized.

They reached the intersection with the main road, and Renbourne rapped on the roof of the carriage. "Time to tell the driver that we are going to Scotland."

She looked at him. "No."

As the carriage slowed to a stop, he turned to her in surprise. "I thought that we had agreed Scotland was a better choice."

"You said that, not I." Her eyes narrowed. "I have seen maps. London is closer, and in all ways better."

He frowned. "London can be a painful place, Meriel."

"I can bear it."

She waited tensely, thinking that if he dismissed her opinion out of hand, she would throw her shoes at him. She had no gift for being told what to do.

But he said, "Very well. You're right that in most ways, London is preferable." Leaning out of the window, he called to the driver, "Head for the London road."

Satisfied, Meriel leaned back in her seat. Renbourne listened very well. A good trait in a future husband.

Chapter 33

Blessed by fine, steady winds, Kyle's chartered ship made swift progress back to Britain. He'd be home before Dominic expected him.

Constancia had been buried in a quiet churchyard beside an orange tree, so the blossoms would sweeten her resting place. Her namesake doves, *las palomas,* cooed from the bell tower as the coffin was lowered into the earth. Teresa had wept for her mistress, but Kyle had watched dry-eyed. He'd already shed his tears for his wife.

Teresa chose to stay in Spain and return to her native town. Kyle left her with a purse of gold that had rounded the girl's eyes and would provide her with a handsome dowry if she found a young man to her liking. Then, more alone than he had ever been in his life, Kyle took ship for his homeland.

He spent much of his time standing in the ship's bow and watching the wheeling gulls as his mind returned again to Cádiz. Would he ever see Spain again? He'd liked what little he'd seen, but guessed that the memories would be too painful to ever allow another visit.

Even to himself, he could not describe his emotions. Sorrow, of course, for that would always be with him. But mostly he felt empty. Hollow as a bubble that would blow away in the first breeze.

The knowledge that Lady Meriel Grahame awaited was a welcome anchor. The unfortunate girl could never be to him what Constancia had been, but she needed a husband to look out for her, and to administer her inheritance with a care no hireling could provide. Though her uncle thought that marriage and perhaps children might cure her disordered wits, Kyle suspected that was wishful thinking. However, he had promised to do his best by the girl, and he would, unless Dominic had failed in his role.

But the substitution should have gone smoothly—how much could go wrong in a quiet place like Warfield? Dominic was thoroughly competent when he chose to be, and he'd wanted the scheme to succeed at least as much as Kyle did.

A gull screamed by no more than a dozen feet away. Remembering the bread he'd brought from his breakfast, Kyle broke off pieces and tossed them into the wind. The swift, greedy birds caught the morsels before they could touch the sea.

He had debated whether to reveal his marriage to anyone back home, but decided against it. Not because he was ashamed of his love for Constancia—never that. But knowing that people would gossip or make rude jokes about his marriage to a courtesan many years his senior was abhorrent. Such talk was unworthy of her memory.

To the world, Lady Meriel would be the first and only Lady Maxwell. It was enough that Kyle had loved Constancia, and she had known it.

Chapter 34

By the time they reached Mayfair, Dominic was wishing he'd argued Meriel out of coming to London. The long journey was hard on her to begin with, for she was unused to spending days trapped in a small, jarring coach, and the need for haste meant that stops were few and brief.

But London was far worse than the extra miles to Scotland would have been. The city always assaulted Dominic's senses when he returned after a spell in the country, and this time the rank odors and clamorous noise seemed infinitely worse because he was imagining how Meriel must feel. As soon as they reached the fringes of the city, she withdrew into a corner of the coach, face pale and her body knotted in a way that said she did not want to be touched. Conditions improved somewhat when they entered cleaner, more fashionable Mayfair, but it was still London and stressful.

He forced himself not to fuss over Meriel, but he could not dismiss a deep fear that she would break under all the strain she had experienced recently. If that happened, she might retreat to her private world so far that no one, not even he, could reach her.

It would have been so much easier if he had fallen in love with a normal, boring girl. The trouble was that such girls were...boring.

He'd thought hard about where to stay in the city. Though his valet, Clement, should be back from the country, Dominic's rooms were no place to take an unmarried young lady. A quiet, respectable hotel seemed a better choice, until the sight of Hyde Park gave him an idea.

Stopping the coach, he gave the driver a new address. As he settled in the vehicle again, he explained, "I just realized that we can probably stay with some friends of mine, Lord and Lady Kimball. I don't believe they've left for the country yet."

Meriel tensed even more. "Fashionable people?"

He shook his head. "They're both painters, and they have the artists' tolerance of unconventional situations. I can't think of a household in London that you would find more congenial. They even have quite a nice garden, by London standards."

She relaxed a little. "Why do you know painters so well?"

How did one explain the spark of mutual enjoyment that was friendship? It was as mysterious in its way as romantic love, though thankfully more common. Sticking with the facts, he replied, "Lady Kimball—Rebecca—is a well-known portrait artist. A lady I once knew was sitting for a portrait and asked me to keep her company." As an idle young man about town, Dominic had plenty of time to indulge such requests, particularly since the lady who asked was a widow with whom he'd been having an amiable affair.

"My friend and Rebecca got into a conversation about the pose and I wandered off, ending up in Kenneth's—that is, Lord Kimball's—studio. He was a soldier—a real one, not a mere pretender, like me. He's famous for his pictures of war, and the consequences of war." Dominic thought back to the moment he'd entered the studio, and been stopped in his tracks by the almost completed painting on Kimball's easel. That was the day he discovered the power of art.

Shaking off the memory, he said, "Kenneth was painting a scene from Waterloo, and that started us talking. I was a very junior cavalry officer while he was captain of a company of the Rifle Brigade, but we were both there, which created an immediate bond. He'd commanded enough young officers like me to understand how I'd been affected—probably better than I did. By the time my friend's portrait was done, Kenneth and Rebecca had adopted me as a sort of little brother. For years I've run tame around their house. They will not be shocked to find us on their doorstep."

Meriel nodded slowly. "They sound...comfortable." And clearly she was in need of comfort, though she didn't look as if she expected to find any.

"The knocker is up, so they haven't left town yet," Dominic said as the carriage halted in front of a handsome corner house. "This place used to belong to Rebecca's father, Sir Anthony Seaton, president of the Royal Academy. Have you heard of him?"

Meriel nodded. Sir Anthony, charmingly arrogant, would be gratified to know that even a total recluse who paid no attention to the world knew his name.

"When Kenneth and Rebecca married, Sir Anthony gave them this large house, and bought the smaller one next door for himself and his wife," Dominic explained. "A door was cut through on the ground floor so the two families can wander back and forth but still have privacy. I don't know another household like it."

Though Dominic had intended to go into Kimball House alone to explain the situation, Meriel climbed out of the carriage after him. No stockings, but she'd slipped on her shoes. Pale, dressed like a servant, and looking as if she would shatter at a touch, she was an odd sight even in London.

No sooner had he and Meriel been admitted by the maid than a small boy shot through the entrance hall. "Uncle Dominic!"

With a grin, Dominic swooped the five-year-old over his head before setting the child back on his feet. "What happened to saying hello before attacking?" he laughed. Turning to Meriel, he said, "Meet the Honorable Michael Seaton Wilding."

To the boy, he said, "Please pay your respects to Lady Meriel Grahame, who has done me the honor to agree to become my wife."

As the boy bowed, a light voice from the steps accused, "Uncle Dominic, you didn't wait for me to grow up."

He glanced up and saw a red-haired girl of eight coming down the stairs, her small body swaddled in a paint-marked smock. "I'm sorry, Antonia," he said apologetically. "But I feared that I would pine for you for the next ten years, and then you would break my heart by refusing to marry me anyhow."

"Very likely." The little girl curtsied gracefully. "Welcome, Lady Meriel."

Next to appear was Rebecca Wilding herself, wearing a smock with almost as much paint as her daughter's. "Dominic, how lovely to see you. It's been too long. Did I hear something about an almost wife?" Her eyes widened when she saw Meriel, the lust of a fascinated painter shining in the hazel depths.

As a hound ambled in and leaned against Dominic, the last human member of the family came down the stairs, burly as a stevedore and smelling faintly of turpentine. "Quite a commotion," Kenneth Wilding observed as he scanned the increasingly crowded hall. "What am I missing?"

By the time all of the introductions were performed, two cats had also materialized, and Meriel looked ready to faint. Dominic put a protective hand on the back of her waist as he considered the best way to proceed.

Meriel solved the problem by straightening to her full height. "Lady Kimball, would you mind terribly if I visit your garden?" Her ironic gaze went to Dominic. "This will be much easier to explain if I'm not present."

Not turning a hair, Rebecca said, "Antonia, take Lady Meriel to the garden, and then leave her in peace. Michael, back upstairs to your lessons."

Meriel and Antonia left, the dog and one of the cats, a large gray tabby, pattering behind. When the adults were alone, Kenneth remarked, "There's obviously quite a story behind this. Do tell us what is going on, Dominic."

"Gladly, though I ask that you not tell anyone else, not even Sir Anthony and Lady Seaton." Dominic accompanied his friends into the drawing room at the back of the house. After they took seats, he gave a terse summary of Meriel's background, how he'd come to meet her, and the reasons why a swift marriage was essential. He concluded with, "This is a great deal to ask, but would you be able to let us stay here one or two nights, until I can make the arrangements for the wedding?"

Kenneth frowned. "Or course you're welcome, but are you sure about this?"

"'Marry in haste, repent at leisure,'" Dominic quoted wryly. "The situation is not ideal, but I'm sure I want to marry her, and I certainly can't allow her uncle to commit her to an asylum again." The memory of her tied to the restraint chair sent a shudder through him that was probably more convincing than his words.

Rebecca and Kenneth exchanged a swift glance. Accord reached, he said, "You must be married here. A wedding in the home of a lord always appears respectable, and it sounds as if you need all the decorum you can get."

"I didn't mean to involve you so closely," Dominic said, startled. "If Lord Grahame chooses to publicly accuse me of seducing his mentally disturbed niece, you could be involved in a nasty scandal."

"We've been boringly well behaved for much too long," Rebecca said blandly. "The ceremony should take place day after tomorrow, I think. Tomorrow is too soon to arrange a proper wedding."

Dominic frowned. "A very small wedding is best. I don't want Meriel strained any further than she is already."

"I understand," Rebecca said reassuringly. "But even if Kenneth and I and perhaps the children are the only guests, there should be some sense of celebration. Marriage is one of life's most important undertakings, so a wedding should not be a sad, shabby affair." She slanted a warm, private glance at her husband. "Believe me, in later years you will both be glad to look back on a day that was special."

Dominic nodded slowly. "You're right,

Rebecca. Meriel has been deprived of so much—she deserves a chance to be a bride. Besides, I'm not sure I could make all the arrangements by tomorrow. The special license, engaging a minister, the marriage settlements..." He started a mental list that included stopping by his rooms for clothing. Marrying Kyle's bride while wearing Kyle's own garments would add insult to injury.

Rising from her chair, Rebecca crossed to the windows at the back of the house, which overlooked the garden. "Will Lady Meriel let me paint her, do you think?"

Dominic set aside his mental list and joined her at the window. The small but pleasant garden had one tree at the far end, with a wooden bench round the trunk. Eyes closed, Meriel sat with her back against the tree. The Kimball hound lay at her feet, while the gray tabby dozed on her lap. He was glad to see that she had regained a little color.

"She might be willing," he replied. "But not on this visit, I think. She's having enough trouble enduring the city."

"Rebecca and Sir Anthony and I may have to draw lots to determine who paints her first," Kenneth observed with amusement. "She has an irresistible ethereal quality."

"I can see her as Daphne," his wife murmured. "Just beginning to turn into a laurel tree to escape being ravished by Apollo."

"I think Keats, myself," Dominic remarked.

"'La Belle Dame Sans Merci?' Perfect," Rebecca said with swift comprehension. Her eyes became hazy with inner vision. "Spun glass with a core of pure steel. A silver maiden in a primeval forest, surrounded by enchanted beasts."

"Later, my love." Kenneth put a firm hand on his wife's shoulder. "What the girl needs now is a refuge, not a mythic painting."

Snapping immediately back to reality, Rebecca said, "Do you think she'd mind if I went out and spoke with her?"

"If she minds, you'll probably know soon enough." Dominic smiled wryly. "Though I'm sure the only person she's bitten has been my father."

Rebecca's eyes filled with laughter. "I think I shall like Lady Meriel." Stripping off her painter's smock, she left the drawing room.

Dominic began to discuss logistics with Kenneth, grateful for the impulse that had led him to this safe haven. Even if Grahame thought to seek his niece in London instead of Gretna Green, he'd never find them in this private home. Two more days and they'd be husband and wife, and Meriel would be safe.

Safe, and his.

Street noise was a constant background hum in London, and Meriel didn't realize she had company until a soft feminine voice asked, "May I join you?"

Ashamed of her earlier weakness, Meriel spent a moment collecting herself so she would not disgrace Dominic in front of his friends. Luckily, a garden and a purring cat were most therapeutic. She opened her eyes. Lady Kimball's light was opalescent, many-layered, and sparked with changeable colors. "Of course, Lady Kimball. Forgive my rudeness in bolting out here."

"London is overwhelming for anyone who grew up in the country." Lady Kimball seated herself on the tree bench to Meriel's right. In her mid-thirties, she wasn't much taller than Meriel, with untidily knotted auburn hair and an air of imperturbable calm. She glanced at the sleeping hound. "Horatio has a taken a remarkable liking to you, and I can only assume that you mesmerized the Gray Ghost, the cat in your lap."

"I like animals." Meriel stroked the old cat's soft fur, wondering if Roxana and Ginger were pining for her. With luck, she would be home within the week. But first, she must learn to be strong. There was nothing very attractive about a female who could not manage the simplest aspects of life.

Lady Kimball leaned over to scratch Horatio, who moaned with canine bliss. "If you don't object, the wedding will be held here the day after tomorrow."

Meriel nodded, relieved. "I would like the privacy of that, Lady Kimball."

"Call me Rebecca." Leaning back against the tree trunk, the older woman said pensively, "I became involved in a scandal when I was a girl, and for years after I lived in this house as a recluse. It was very hard to emerge from solitude and reenter society."

Meriel cocked her head to one side. "How did you manage?"

"Very badly. Kenneth had to drag me, kicking and screaming, to my first ball."

"I see why he and Dominic are friends," Meriel said dryly.

"They share a certain directness," the other woman agreed. "Even with Kenneth at my side, my first venture into the fashionable world was ghastly. People stared, whispered behind my back, even insulted me to my face. But Kenneth's friends accepted me for his sake, and soon I was glad to have rejoined the world. Though my attic studio was safe, it lacked variety."

So because Kenneth's friends had helped Rebecca, she was now doing the same for another outsider. Generous of her to try to make Meriel feel like less of a freak, though the situations were hardly the same. Meriel said wistfully, "I think my journey to the world will be much longer than yours."

"Longer, and surely harder," the other woman said quietly. "But with determination and the right companion, any journey is possible. You chose well with Dominic. I've never known a kinder, more accepting man, except for Kenneth."

Rebecca was right—Dominic had been saintly in his patience and understanding. Too saintly, perhaps, for a female who was more pagan than lady.

Interrupting her thoughts, Rebecca asked, "Is there anything you would like for your wedding, or any questions you'd like to ask?"

Understanding what wasn't said, Meriel replied, "Are you going to offer me a lesson on my marital duties? A very embarrassed general in Shropshire attempted that."

"No lessons unless you ask for them," Rebecca promised, her gaze shrewd. "But I would like to offer you a gown to be married in. You and I are near the same size, and I have something that should suit you very well."

"Thank you." Meriel felt a sting of tears; the last days had left her emotions scraped raw and too easily affected. She hated feeling so vulnerable. "You're very good to a mad stranger."

"You appear saner than half the painters I know. Not that that's difficult!" Rebecca rose to her feet. "Stay out here as long as you like. When you're ready, you'll have a nice quiet room at the back of the house."

"Thank you," Meriel said again, wishing she were more eloquent. To her own surprise, she reached out to touch the other woman's hand. "I'm glad that Dominic brought me here."

Rebecca took her hand in a warm, turpentine-scented clasp. "I hope we see more of you. Dominic is almost a member of the family, and that means you are, too." Rebecca's gaze sharpened as she noticed the fading mehndi bracelet on Meriel's wrist. "What's this?"

"Mehndi. They are temporary designs painted in henna, very common in India and other Eastern countries."

Eyes bright as a girl's, Rebecca dropped onto

380

the bench again. "How fascinating! Please, tell me more. Do the patterns have special meanings? Is it possible to get the henna here in London?"

With a smile, Meriel began answering her hostess's questions. It was good to have something to offer in return for all she was being given.

Chapter 35

Dominic was relieved to see that Meriel looked almost her normal self when she returned from the garden, though obviously she was tired. With only a brief glance for him, she requested a light supper in her room so she could go to bed early.

Tired himself and not wanting to disrupt the household routine any more than necessary, Dominic also excused himself not long after dinner. But before going to his room, he stopped to check on Meriel.

She called permission at his knock, and he entered to find her perched on a window seat, legs drawn up and arms locked around her knees as she gazed into the long summer twilight. The gray tabby had accompanied her, and was daintily finishing off the last of Meriel's supper.

"I hope you ate something before the Gray Ghost took over your plate." Dominic kissed the top of Meriel's head, then sat in a chair by the window seat. Her bare toes peeped from beneath the hem of her dress.

"The Gray Ghost and I made a bargain," she said without looking at him. "I got the first half of the meal, and he gets the second half."

"You're feeling better?"

She nodded, her gaze on the urban garden, or perhaps the jumbled rooftops of Mayfair. "But my life has changed so much that sometimes I wonder if I'm dreaming."

He studied her cool profile. "Are you sorry for the changes?"

She was silent for a long time. "I suppose not. Much has been gained. But I was happy before you came, not knowing or caring what I missed. Would I have been better off staying as I was? I cannot say."

He winced. Though in general he appreciated honesty, it hurt that she was so ambivalent about having him in her life. Trying not to sound defensive, he said, "Change would have come sooner or later. Lord Amworth was all that ever stood between you and the asylum, and he's older and in poorer health than Lord Grahame."

"Perhaps Warfield was the dream. If so, it was a happy one."

"Are you unhappy now?"

She shivered. "I feel...suspended."

As much for his comfort as for hers, he stood and lifted her from the window seat, then sat in the chair again with her across his lap. She exhaled softly and settled against him, her head on his shoulder. As the light faded, he stroked her back, reassured by her weight and warmth and familiar scent.

Knowing that it must be said, he murmured, "It's not too late to change your mind about marriage if you truly don't wish it, Meriel. Other arrangements can be made to keep you away from your uncle. Rebecca's parents are about to leave for their summer house in the Lake District. Rebecca said you could go with them, and stay for the next several months. It's a wild, quiet place. I think you'd like it there."

Her slim body tensed, and the silence stretched so long that he was sure she would take this opportunity to back out. Instead, she asked in a flat little voice, "Are you having second thoughts now that you have seen how ill-suited I am to be a wife?"

"Good God, no!" he exclaimed. "What gave you that idea?"

"I have caused you a great deal of trouble. Now that we are here in London, it must be obvious that I will never be 'normal.'" She tilted her head back, her eyes unreadable in the dim light. "Society says that a gentleman who proposes marriage is not allowed to change his mind—only ladies have that privilege. A stupid rule. I release you of all obligations. You wished to rescue me, and you have. Being a gentleman should not cost you more than it already has."

His pulse began hammering. "I want you not from obligation, but from love, Meriel. I just had to be sure that you are marrying me of your own free will."

Her mouth twisted with patent disbelief.

Horrified by the realization that they were a hairsbreadth from splitting apart, he kissed her hard, wanting to burn away her doubts. After a startled moment, her mouth opened under his and she responded with fierce hunger. As desire scorched through him, he realized that *this* was what they had needed.

They had not made love since the night she'd been rescued from the asylum. On the journey, they had occupied separate rooms for propriety's sake, and because he had not wanted to burden her with physical demands when she was under so much stress.

But passion was healing, a way to renew the fraying intimacy. He felt her coming alive, kissing back, her nails digging into his shoulders.

As the kiss became deeper and deeper, he slid his hand up her leg, under the skirt of her borrowed dress. She opened her knees so that he could skim the silky skin inside her thighs. When he touched the moist, heated folds of hidden flesh, she gasped. He probed more deeply, caressing until her hips began rolling, grinding provocatively into his lap. Feverishly he swept her up and laid her across the scarlet counterpane.

Then, urgent, heedless of subtlety, he unbuttoned his trousers and mounted her, yanking aside skirts and petticoats so he could thrust into her hotly welcoming body. She sucked in her breath when he entered, then wrapped arms and legs around him so their plunging bodies would stay locked together.

Their coupling was swift and feral, a fury of the blood that fused them into one. When he felt her convulsing, he captured her mouth so they absorbed their cries in each other. He poured himself into her, then subsided, shaking and dizzy, as he wondered at the madness that had overcome them both.

Panting for breath, he rolled onto his side. "Do you still doubt that I want you?"

She gave a soft laugh and touched his cheek. "No, Dominic."

As he heard the satisfaction in her voice, he realized that she had needed to know what power she had over him. Under her air of fragility was great strength, and for many years she had been master of her own life within the confines of Warfield.

But lately she'd been buffeted by forces beyond her control, and that had left her off balance. She needed reassurance that she was not a helpless victim. Tenderly he kissed her temple, thinking how lucky he was that reassuring her was so richly rewarding.

The subject of withdrawing from the marriage was not mentioned again.

The morning began well, with a visit to the Kimballs' solicitor, chosen because Dominic wanted no part of the family lawyer who had revealed Amworth's plans to Lord Grahame. The solicitor, a shrewd-eyed man named Carlton, promised to immediately draw up documents to keep Meriel's fortune under her control so they could be signed that afternoon at Kimball House.

Procuring a special license at Doctor's Commons proved simple, if time-consuming, and the vicar of the local parish was willing and able to perform the ceremony. Dominic's last stop at his rooms had the bonus of finding his valet, Clement, who had just returned from visiting his sick mother, now much improved.

It was a relief to confide the events of the last weeks to Clement, who was as much friend as servant. Though the valet rolled his eyes eloquently several times during the narrative, he efficiently packed Dominic's clothing and wished his master a pleasant wedding day. Dominic considered inviting Clement to the ceremony but decided against it. Meriel didn't need more strangers around her. The valet could join him later.

Dominic returned to Kimball House to find that Meriel had become a household favorite. Besides playing with the children and keeping Rebecca company in the studio, she'd used weeds, garden flowers, and an ancient, paint-encrusted pot to create an arrangement. When Rebecca saw it, she remarked, "Meriel has the eye of an artist."

"A painter in blossom and branch," Dominic agreed. Now that he'd learned to appreciate Meriel's originality, he loved her creations.

Late in the afternoon, Carlton arrived with the draft marriage settlements. At a meeting in the study, the lawyer explained the provisions to Meriel. Kenneth also attended as a general advocate for Meriel's interests. Dominic didn't want there to ever be any suggestion that he had taken advantage of her in any way.

Faced by three earnest men, Meriel listened to the proposed settlements with a vaguely unfocused expression that worried Dominic. She seemed to have withdrawn from sheer boredom, and didn't really grasp the importance of what was being decided.

He should have known better. After Carlton's summary, she scanned the document, then calmly ripped it into pieces. As the men stared, she said, "The provisions for children seemed reasonable. Retain them. As for the rest, draw up a settlement in which Renbourne and I share equally in responsibility for Warfield, and have equal access to all moneys. Neither of us may do anything drastic, such as selling off land or investments, without the consent of the other."

Carlton's jaw dropped. "That is a very radical arrangement."

Meriel's delicate brows arched. "But surely not illegal?"

"Not if properly drawn," the lawyer admitted.

"Then do it." Meriel got to her feet. Wearing a simple blue morning gown of Rebecca's, she was every inch an aristocrat. "If I die before my husband, he is heir to all I own. If we both die without children, my fortune goes back to whence it came—the land to my mother's family, the bulk of the money to my father's people."

Dominic stammered, "B-but you wanted to have all of your holdings in trust, so that I would not be able to misuse your fortune."

"Your idea, not mine," she said coolly. "I said I would rather be your mistress than your wife, but I have never distrusted your honesty." She inclined her head. "Gentlemen." Then she turned and left the study, her long flaxen braid swaying gently.

Dominic, still stunned, saw that Kenneth was shaking with silent laughter. Carlton took off his gold-rimmed spectacles and polished them with his handkerchief. "A remarkable young lady, Mr. Renbourne. One who knows her own mind. While her settlement requirements are most unusual, one cannot say they are unreasonable."

Grinning, Kenneth said, "You're marrying a sylph of steel, Dominic. One can see the blood of Norman conquerors in her veins." Gaze becoming unfocused, he picked up a pencil and began sketching on a piece of torn settlement paper. "*That's* the way to paint her—as a Norman chatelaine on the castle walls, defending herself and her people against siege while her noble husband is away. Fragile but indomitable as she brandishes a sword to rally her men-at-arms."

Dominic rolled his eyes, knowing he'd get no more sense out of Kenneth for a while. But even though Meriel had made him look like an idiot in front of the other men, her gesture warmed him. She wanted them to be equal partners. Not a common arrangement, but very fair, and exactly what he would have chosen.

Better yet, she had said in as many words that she trusted him. Someday, God willing, she would love him as well.

Chapter 36

Kyle felt a curious sense of unreality when he arrived back in London. Everything seemed exactly the same, almost as if he hadn't left. Yet at the same time, he felt as if he had been away for years and changed beyond recognition.

Shaking off his disorientation, he decided that the first order of business was to visit his brother's rooms. They had agreed on several possible methods of establishing contact on Kyle's return, depending on how matters went at Warfield. First and easiest would be if Dominic had fulfilled his mission and returned to London.

If that was the case, Dominic had only to brief Kyle on the events of his visit, and Kyle would proceed from there. A swift wedding, he presumed, because Lady Meriel's uncle Grahame would return from the Continent in another fortnight or so.

If Dominic was still at Warfield, he should have sent a message to his man Clement. If the valet was still in the country, Kyle would have to travel to Shropshire and secretly communicate with his brother, or go to ground until Dominic returned to London. Certainly it would be impossible to change places at Warfield; even the least observant person would notice if Dominic turned into Kyle overnight. Some time must elapse to blur the differences between them.

Kyle suspected that Dominic had become bored with life at Warfield and returned to London by now. If so, the deception was over, with no one the wiser.

Impatient to finish the business, he traveled to Dominic's lodgings. As he waited in the dim hallway, he was glad to hear footsteps responding to his knock on the door. At least one of the men was back in London.

Clement opened the door. Arching his brows, the valet asked, "Did you forget something, sir? If you don't hurry, you'll be late for your own wedding."

Kyle froze as a premonition of disaster struck him. "What wedding?"

Clement looked closer, and paled. "Good God, Lord Maxwell!"

He tried to slam the door, but he was too late. Kyle forced his way into the flat, demanding, "Who is Dominic marrying?"

Poker-faced, the valet backed slowly into the small drawing room. "I misspoke, my lord. I was not expecting to see you."

"That's for damned sure!" He advanced on Clement, expression thunderous. "He's marrying Lady Meriel Grahame, isn't he? *Isn't he?*"

Despite Kyle's premonition, the flicker of acknowledgment on Clement's face was a numbing blow. How could Dominic have betrayed him so treacherously?

Yet it made perfect sense—Dominic had always resented being the younger son, with no property and only limited income and status. Marrying the mad Lady Meriel would set him up in style for life. Instead of having to settle for a modest estate, he was now master of a fortune equal to the Wrexham inheritance. It was all so *logical*.

And all Kyle's fault, for being bloody fool enough to trust his brother. He spat out, "Where and when?"

The valet shook his head, refusing to answer. The rage that had been building since Kyle had learned of Constancia's fatal illness exploded. He slammed the slightly built Clement against the wall and locked his hands around his throat with bruising force. "Tell me, or by God, I'll choke it out of you! Where is Dominic marrying her?"

Clement gasped, "A-at Kimball House, but there's no use trying to stop the ceremony." His frightened gaze went to the mantel clock. "It will be over before you can get there. You're too late."

Swearing, Kyle released the valet and headed for the door. It might be too late to stop the wedding, but there was still time to break his brother's neck.

Rebecca had been right—it was worth the extra effort to make the wedding special. Wearing a gown of ivory silk, with her incredible hair falling free under a fine veil and a chaplet of fresh flowers, Meriel was so beautiful that Dominic's heart hurt. She entered the drawing room carrying a bouquet of roses and trailing ivy, her small feet bare and elegant and utterly enchanting.

Decorated with massed flowers, the room had become a place of celebration. Rebecca and Kenneth were the attendants, with their children and Rebecca's parents as the only guests, but it was enough. Meriel would not look back on her wedding day and feel that she had been deprived. Nor would Dominic.

Suppressing the painful knowledge that he was about to drive the last nails into the coffin of his relationship with his brother, he took Meriel's hand and turned to the vicar, who stood with his back to the windows. The vicar had a warm smile for them, and for the Gray Ghost, who watched with interest from the sofa. In a sonorous voice, he began, "Dearly beloved, we are gathered together here in the sight of God..."

The stately, familiar words flowed over Dominic, bringing him a sense of peace. He and Meriel belonged together. When she said her vows in a soft, clear voice, it was hard to remember the wild girl who had fled his presence when they first met.

Dominic's mind went blank when the vicar

asked for the ring. He'd purchased one the day before, hadn't he? Where was it? Before panic could set in, Kenneth produced the ring, a twinkle in his eyes. Dominic was lucky to have him for a friend.

He'd always assumed that if he married, his brother would be his best man....

Suppressing the thought, he slid the ring on Meriel's finger. She gave him a clear, green-eyed glance. His exquisite little pagan, enchanting and stubborn, mysterious and magical. He uttered a private prayer that he would always be worthy of her.

The rest of the service was a haze, until the vicar said, "I pronounce that they be man and wife together," and gave the final blessing.

After Dominic kissed his bride, the guests crowded forward, laughing and offering congratulations. Dominic accepted them, giddy with happiness. Meriel was his, to love, honor, and protect. Together they could face whatever might come.

He barely noticed a commotion in the hallway, until the doors flew open and Kyle burst into the drawing room, hair wild and expression dangerous. Only Dominic was looking in his direction, and for one endless, excruciating moment, Kyle's raging gaze met Dominic's. Then he stormed down the long room, shouting, "You *bastard!*"

His curse cut through the laughter, and the startled guests spun around to stare at the interloper. Meriel inhaled sharply, looking from Kyle to Dominic and back again. The Kimballs and Seatons did the same. For anyone who had never seen them together, the resemblance was downright eerie.

With a feeling of numb inevitability, Dominic gently set Meriel aside and advanced toward his twin. "This isn't what you think."

Kyle's answer was an incoherent growl, and a fist that smashed into his brother's jaw. Dominic didn't even try to avoid it. The impact spun him around, but he welcomed the blow. If only pain could wash away the crushing guilt.

"Enough!" Broad and formidable, Kenneth Wilding was on Kyle before he could strike again. Twisting one arm behind Kyle's back with a strength that immobilized the younger man, he ordered, "Give Dominic a chance to explain."

Kyle struggled to free himself, then gasped when Kenneth increased the pressure to the agonizing point just short of dislocating the shoulder. "What is there to explain?" he said bitterly, ignoring everyone except Dominic. "You've always despised me for the crime of being born first, and now you've got your revenge. *Damn* you!"

The devastation in Kyle's eyes paralyzed Dominic, reflecting back to combine with his own anguish. All he could do was say numbly, "I'm sorry, Kyle, but for Meriel's sake, there was no other way."

"You bloody hypocrite!" Snarling obscenities, Kyle tried to break free again.

Kenneth stopped that by jerking the pinioned

394

arm upward. "I don't care how upset you are, I'll have no such language in front of my wife and children! If you want to talk to your brother civilly, fine. If not, get out of my house."

A pulse throbbed in Kyle's forehead, but he stopped fighting. "I never thought you'd stoop this low, Dominic," he said in a shaking voice. "Christ! I'd been hoping that maybe we could be friends again, and all the while you were betraying me." His mouth twisted. "So clever. Not only did you get the pleasure of seducing my betrothed wife, but in the process you got the money and power you've always wanted. And to think I was fool enough to trust you merely because you're my *brother*."

"There was no malice in this, I swear." Dominic halted, achingly aware that it would be useless to explain that he loved Meriel and had needed to move swiftly to protect her. Kyle was so enraged that all he could see was the fact of betrayal. Any reasons Dominic offered would seem like cowardly excuses.

Taking a firm hold of Dominic's arm, Meriel said sharply, "You much mistake the matter, Lord Maxwell. I would never have married you, so you have no right to blame Dominic for stealing your bride."

For the first time, Kyle looked at her. He blinked, startled, as if he didn't quite recognize the woman he had intended to marry. Then he turned his furious gaze back to his brother. Meriel no longer mattered—it was Dominic who had committed the unforgivable crime. "I'm sorry, Kyle," he whispered again.

"It's time you left, Lord Maxwell," Rebecca said crisply. "I suggest that after you calm down, you discuss this matter with Dominic, but not before."

Kenneth released Kyle's arm, then escorted him from the drawing room. Rigid to the breaking point, Kyle left without looking back.

Dominic knew he should do something—anything—to break the frozen silence. This whole ghastly mess was his fault. But he was numbed by an unholy mixture of his own and his brother's pain. Knowing that Kyle had wanted to try rebuilding their relationship added an extra dimension of torment.

Meriel guided him to the nearest chair. As she pushed him into the seat, she ordered, "Leave us."

Silently the other guests obeyed. Even the cat left the room.

When they were alone, Meriel embraced Dominic, cradling his head to her breasts. "I'm sorry," she said quietly as she stroked the back of his neck. "I did not really understand how badly your brother would take news of our marriage."

Dominic wrapped his arms around her, shaking and chilled to the bone. "Kyle and I have been estranged for years, but there was always a basic trust. I have broken that, and he will never forgive me." Kyle had never been very good at forgiveness—he'd left that to Dominic.

"You broke faith with him to keep faith

with me. That took a great and terrible courage." She rested her cheek against his hair. "Thank you, my husband."

He closed his eyes, concentrating on her blessed warmth and his own breathing. In, out. In, out. This was worse than if Kyle had died, for death would be devastating but relatively simple. A mere matter of losing part of his soul. This savage rupture, a nightmare of anguish and betrayal, would permanently scar both Kyle and himself.

Could he have done anything differently, perhaps hidden Meriel somewhere safe until after Kyle returned? His brother would still have been furious, but it would not have been as bad as learning about the marriage in such a shattering way.

The sickening image of Meriel tied to the chair at Bladenham flashed through Dominic's mind. He could not have risked that happening again. The danger from Grahame had been very real. Her uncle had been a soldier. If he'd run them down with a magistrate at his back and a dueling pistol in his hand, it might have ended with Dominic dead and Meriel locked in some hellish asylum, dying by inches.

Bleakly he accepted that he could not have risked acting differently, not when Meriel's safety and sanity were at sake. He'd made his choice, and now he must live with the consequences. At least, thank God, Meriel trusted him enough to know that he hadn't acted from the base motives Kyle had accused him of.

Life went on. Eventually, this pain would diminish to a bearable level. It would be harder for Kyle, who didn't have a Meriel, and who had so recently suffered some other great grief. That knowledge was another slash of the blade that had already left Dominic's heart bleeding.

But he could not sit here clinging to Meriel like a terrified child forever. He released his grip and looked up her. She was regarding him gravely, the window behind her transforming her flaxen hair and white veil into a nimbus of light. She looked like an angel, though he knew her well enough to see the steel beneath the silk.

Delicately she skimmed his cheek with butterfly fingertips. "I used to dream that I had a twin sister," she said softly. "A sister soul who would be my best friend, who would always love and understand me. I never thought of the dark side of being twin-born— the ability to devastate each other."

He sighed. "You and I shall have to be each other's best friends, my love."

Seeing that he had regained his control, she smiled and gave him a light, sweet kiss. "Aren't we now?"

He managed to smile back. "You are worth any price, Meriel."

"I'm glad you realize that," she said demurely. "Now, my husband, we will partake of the wedding breakfast with our good friends, so they will forget the unpleasantness and remember only the joy. Then we shall return home to Warfield."

He got to his feet and pulled her into a hug. "I like it when you're imperious."

"Then in the future you should be a very happy man."

Despite his mood, he had to laugh. Arm around his bride, he headed from the drawing room. Perhaps someday, God willing, Kyle would listen to reason, though Dominic wasn't counting on it. Even if that never happened, at least he had Meriel.

Kyle didn't know how long he walked blindly around London, unaware of his surroundings as his pulse hammered *betrayed, betrayed, betrayed. And by Dominic, whom he had never imagined could be his enemy.*

His mind finally cleared on Westminster Bridge when he leaned on the parapet and stared down at the rushing waters of the Thames. In a distant part of his mind, he realized that he was actually thinking about jumping.

His hands tightened on the stone at the horrifying awareness that he had fallen so low. Think how satisfied Dominic would be—with Kyle dead, he would be the next Earl of Wrexham, and one of the richest men in England.

Kyle turned grimly from the river. He'd be damned if he'd let Dominic have Wrexham. Besides, with his luck, he'd probably be pulled ignominiously from the water by one of the busy Thames riverboats.

The emptiness that filled him since Constancia's death had expanded to a whole new dimension. What would he do with his life now that he no longer had Lady Meriel Grahame to anchor him to the world?

Certainly he must find another bride and get several sons on her so that Dominic would never inherit Wrexham. But courtship would have to wait. It had been possible to imagine a shadow marriage with a witless girl, but the thought of putting a real wife in Constancia's place was unendurable.

He could summon only one frail goal: to return to Dornleigh. It was the least welcoming great house in England, but it was home. Vaguely he remembered that his father and sister had intended to visit Lucia's future in-laws, so with luck he'd have the place to himself, bar a hundred or so servants.

Dornleigh. Odd how the desire to go home survived when all else was gone. He gave thanks for that, for otherwise there would be nothing left.

Chapter 37

"Welcome home!" Jena Ames came out to meet the carriage, greeting Meriel with a hug. "I presume you're now Lady Meriel Renbourne?"

Meriel blinked. She hadn't thought about her new name. "So I am."

Dominic smiled at her with a warmth that sent tingles through interesting places. The

400

return to Shropshire had been more relaxed than the journey to London. She hadn't realized how much mischief one could get into inside a carriage....

"Meriel managed London very well," Dominic said. "I believe I even heard her say, when we were a safe distance from the city, that she might like to visit again."

"But not *soon*," Meriel said austerely. Though she still had her doubts about cities, she had enjoyed Rebecca and Kenneth and their children. She had even come to appreciate the sense of excitement that was as much a part of London as the soot. The next visit to the metropolis would be easier.

Laughing, they entered Holliwell Grange. By the time Jena had ordered a tea tray, the general had appeared from the stables. "So the deed is done," he said jovially. After shaking Dominic's hand, he kissed the bride, smelling not unpleasantly of horse.

Conversation was casual until they'd had tea and currant cakes. Then Jena purposefully set her cup aside. "Lord Grahame raced up to Gretna Green trying to find you, Meriel. Since he failed, he's waiting at Warfield for you two to return."

Meriel nodded. Her uncle would know that she wouldn't stay away from Warfield for long.

"Thank you for the information," Dominic said soberly. "I've wondered what he has been doing."

Jena dropped her gaze, her cheeks coloring. "Kamal has kept us informed."

Apparently matters were progressing between Jena and Kamal. Meriel asked, "The ladies are well?"

"Yes, and much relieved after Kamal told them you'd gone off to marry." Jena glanced at Dominic. "They approve of you."

Meriel saw the faint tightening of her husband's face. He had not referred to the disastrous scene his brother had made at the wedding, but she felt the ache inside him. She wondered if he would ever forgive himself for doing what had to be done.

The general said flatly, "Now what?"

Meriel and Dominic exchanged a glance. They had discussed this on the journey, and agreed that the direct approach would be best. "We plan to ride to Warfield together, and would appreciate your joining us in your capacity as magistrate," she said. "I can pretend to be a completely sane lady for long enough to convince my uncle that his misguided efforts on my behalf are no longer needed."

"I'll come, too," Jena said. "The more supporters Meriel has, the better."

The general nodded. "Grahame is stubborn, but no fool. Once he gets it through his skull that Lady Meriel is normal, your problems are over."

Meriel frowned. "Will speech and good clothing be enough to convince people I'm sane after so many years when I was considered mad?"

"Actually, those things *are* enough. We are judged largely by appearances. If you talk and dress as a lady, by definition you are a lady." Dominic smiled wryly. "And of course you're an heiress, which means that you are charmingly eccentric, not mad."

The others nodded agreement, but Meriel was less sure. It was hard to believe reclaiming her home would be so easy.

After breakfast the next morning, the party set off for Warfield on four of the general's excellent horses. Meriel rode beside Dominic, head high, splendid hair coiled beneath a hat, and expression perfectly composed. Rebecca had given her a riding habit, so she used a sidesaddle and looked every inch a lady. Only someone who knew her well would recognize that she was wound tighter than a clock spring.

When they reached the wrought iron gates of Warfield, Meriel rang the bell. The gatekeeper emerged from the handsome gatehouse at his usual leisurely pace.

Meriel inclined her head. "Good day, Walter."

The old man's jaw dropped in disbelief. "Lady Meriel?"

"Of course." When he continued to stare, she said sweetly, "The gate, please?"

Hastily Walter unlatched the gates and swung them open. The riders came through, then headed up the long drive four abreast. In his head, Dominic could hear the steady rhythm of army marching drums. Appropriate since they rode to battle.

His nerves were taut, though he couldn't imagine any real trouble, not when they had General Ames and the weight of Anglo-Saxon common law on their side. Amazing how much difference a wedding made. Nonetheless, when they approached the house he was relieved to see Grahame stalking down the front steps unarmed. He hadn't forgotten the older man's threats when he threw Dominic out of Warfield.

Lord Grahame's gimlet gaze swept across the riders as they halted. Above him, Mrs. Rector and Mrs. Marks emerged to stand tensely at the top of the wide stone steps.

In a voice of barely suppressed fury, Grahame snapped, "Your gall amazes me, Maxwell. I've been searching all over England for my niece. General Ames, do you know what this young devil has been doing? You can't, or you wouldn't be beside him."

Dominic held his breath as Meriel dismounted gracefully and stood before Grahame, her small figure erect and unyielding as she faced him down. "You should speak to me, Uncle, not my husband and friends."

The blood drained from Grahame's face. "My God, you can talk!"

"Indeed." Meriel looked up at the ladies. "Hello, Mrs. Rector and Mrs. Marks. I hope you have not been too concerned on my behalf."

"We were worried at first," Mrs. Marks admitted. Beside her, Mrs. Rector beamed with delight. The enthralled faces of a dozen servants were visible in the windows above. By evening, everyone in Shropshire would know that Lady Meriel was in complete possession of her faculties.

Grahame stammered, "B-but if you can talk, how come you never did?"

"I had nothing to say." Meriel handed her reins to a wide-eyed footman who came down the steps. Voice edged, she continued, "Nor was I mad. While your intentions were good, I did *not* appreciate being kidnapped and locked up in that vile asylum, nor did I enjoy your threats to my future husband. I trust that nothing so absurd will happen again."

Her uncle said defensively, "Given your behavior, you really can't blame me for assuming you were in need of protection."

Her sardonic glance said that she could indeed blame him, but would graciously refrain. Turning to her companions, she said as casually as if she regularly went riding with friends, "Do please come in for coffee."

Another footman appeared, and the horses were led away as Meriel and company ascended the steps. Dominic took the chance to murmur to her, "Well done! Only a little longer now."

She nodded, tense but well in command of herself and the situation.

Though Grahame's jaw was twitching, he did his best to adjust to the new circumstances. By the time everyone was seated in the large salon, he was able to say with a stiff smile, "I'm sorry for the problems I caused you, Meriel. I...I had thought I was caring for you as my brother would have wished."

Apparently deciding his apology was adequate, Meriel gave her uncle a stunning smile as she stripped off her riding gloves. "I can understand your misapprehensions. We shall speak no more of it. I was fortunate to have two such conscientious guardians."

The awkwardness was broken when Roxana came galloping up to Meriel, tail wagging and almost beside herself with excitement. Meriel knelt for a few moments to assure the excited dog that she truly had come home.

Her gaze on Meriel's wedding ring, Mrs. Marks remarked, "Marriage must agree with you, Mer...Lady Maxwell. I've never seen you look so well."

Meriel exchanged a glance with Dominic as she rose to her feet. This had also been discussed on the return journey. "I am not Lady Maxwell, but Lady Meriel Renbourne. My husband, whom you have come to know and value these last weeks, is Dominic Renbourne, twin brother to Lord Maxwell."

The ladies gasped, and Lord Grahame's jaw dropped. "I beg your pardon?" he said in a dangerous voice. "Wrexham has palmed off a younger son on my niece?"

Smoothly Dominic said, "My father knew nothing of the switch. In fact, he still doesn't. I must write him and my sister tonight." He'd considered writing from London, but decided it would be better to wait until matters were resolved at Warfield.

Mrs. Marks frowned. "How could Wrexham

not know? He and your sister were visitors here for two days!"

"My father's vision is poor, and he expected to see Maxwell," Dominic explained. "Lucia's eyes are younger and keener, and she recognized me immediately, but held her tongue at my request, since the situation was somewhat awkward."

"Awkward indeed," Mrs. Marks said dryly. "I've heard of children amusing themselves by changing places, but never of an adult sending his twin into a courtship."

Dominic offered his most reliable smile, along with the explanation he and Meriel had concocted, half truth and half lie. "There is often a...a special connection between twins. When my brother met Meriel, he had a very strong intuition that she and I would suit. He persuaded me to come in his place for the second, lengthier visit. I agreed with great reluctance because of the deception involved, but Maxwell was most convincing."

"Dominic revealed his true identity very early," Meriel said serenely. "To be honest, I had not been drawn to Lord Maxwell. An estimable man, but not restful. Though they look much the same, Dominic is very different." She gave him a conspicuously doting smile; the minx had the makings of an actress.

Glad to say something that was wholly true, Dominic said, "I was shocked to find myself falling in love with Meriel, but once I did..." He spread his hands in a gesture meant to imply that love conquered all and fate moved in mysterious ways. Though it was a feeble explanation for an outrageous situation, Kyle was unlikely to contradict it. He would look like a fool if he told the truth, and Kyle did not like looking foolish.

Mrs. Rector said admiringly, "What a tale! As fine as any of Mrs. Radcliffe's."

Dominic gave her a sharp glance, thinking he heard irony in her comment. She met his gaze blandly. If she disbelieved his version of events, she kept it to herself.

Grahame still looked indignant that Meriel had ended up with an untitled younger son, but he knew better than to challenge a situation that had been accepted by the ladies, the Ameses, and Meriel herself. In a conciliatory tone, he suggested, "Since the heir to Warfield has married, there should be a celebration for the tenants and villagers."

Mrs. Rector brightened. "Oh, yes. It's a very old family tradition, Meriel."

Knowing how tiring it was for Meriel to play the role of gracious lady, Dominic asked warily, "What kind of celebration?"

"Midsummer Eve is just a few days away. That would be a perfect time for an outdoor feast and bonfire. With luck, Amworth might be well enough to come with his wife, and perhaps your family as well, Renbourne." Grahame's voice turned sardonic. "After all, none of us were fortunate enough to attend the wedding."

Dominic glanced at Meriel. Perhaps because

she had been silent for so long, they found it easy to communicate without words. He arched his brows in question. Since she could easily slip away from such an event if the crowd became overpowering, she nodded her consent. "That would be splendid, if Mrs. Marks and Mrs. Rector agree."

"The choice is Lady Meriel's. Since she no longer needs chaperons or companions, our authority is at an end." Now that Mrs. Marks's initial excitement at Meriel's return had passed, there was anxiety in her eyes. The situation at Warfield had been a godsend for a pair of poor widows.

Meriel said immediately, "You are my family, and Warfield is your home." Her gaze moved from Mrs. Marks to Mrs. Rector. "I hope you will stay here always."

As Mrs. Marks relaxed, Mrs. Rector rose to give Meriel a hug. "Bless you, child." Resuming her seat, she said, "Perhaps we should move to the Dower House, Edith, and give these young people more privacy."

"Such details can be decided later," Dominic said. "Now we must think about the wedding feast, since that is less than a week away."

Two pots of coffee later, all of the plans had been made, mostly by the ladies and Jena. Having been her father's hostess in India, she had a number of practical suggestions for arranging a large gathering on short notice. Invitations would be sent to Dornleigh and Bridgton Abbey. Dominic doubted that his father would come—Wrexham would probably be as furious as Grahame at the change in bride-grooms—but certainly the Renbournes should be invited.

Coffee and planning completed, the Ameses left. As soon as the door closed behind them, Grahame excused himself, ostensibly to attend to correspondence. Dominic suspected that his real desire was to find a quiet place to absorb what had happened. Changing his opinion of his "mad" niece was obviously a painful process.

The ladies withdrew to the morning room for embroidery and a good private gossip, leaving Dominic, Meriel, and the adoring Roxana in the hall. Dominic gave Meriel a quick hug. "You did it, sprite! The battle was won with no blood spilled, and you've been accepted by everyone as mistress of Warfield."

"With the help of my friends." Eyes shining, Meriel ripped off her riding boots and stock-ings. "Finally!"

She yanked out her hairpins and shook loose the primly coiled chignon, then shed her riding jacket and darted down the hall that led to the back of house. Dominic blinked, then took off after her.

Meriel burst into the open air, caroling her delight to the Shropshire skies. Exuberantly she raced down the steps and into the parterre, her flaxen hair flying behind her and Roxana barking at her heels. The London lady had turned back into the wild, magical creature who had first captured Dominic's heart.

As exhilarated as his bride, he followed her along the garden paths, which had grown as familiar as the lines on his own palm. He stayed half a dozen steps behind Meriel, not trying to catch her, enjoying the sight of her swift, supple form.

She finally ran out of energy in a small glade in the wilderness area. Laughing, she collapsed on the soft, flower-strewn grass, heedless of her handsome riding habit. "It's so wonderful to be *home*!"

He dropped onto the grass beside her while Roxana flopped happily on the other side. "Does Warfield seem different to you?"

"Better." Lying on her back, she stretched luxuriantly. "It will be worth leaving sometimes just to have the pleasure of coming back. I think I'd like to travel, someday. Italy. Vienna. The Greek Isles." She laughed suddenly. "And perhaps I'll write a book on how to arrange flowers in ways that almost no one will like or understand!"

"You might start a new fashion." Thinking of another topic that needed discussion, he asked, "How do you feel about children? In the nature of things, they often come quickly after a marriage."

She frowned, her eyes darkening. Dismayed, Dominic realized that she'd had virtually no contact with children for many years, so it might be hard for her to imagine herself as a mother. Hoping she didn't hate the idea of a family too much, he said, "I'm sorry, we should have discussed this before.

If it isn't already too late, there are methods to delay starting a family, if you would prefer that."

She sat up and crossed her legs, expression troubled. "I think I would like to wait a while, but that isn't what bothered me. I...I just remembered a fragment of conversation about having a baby. An argument. But I can't remember when, or who was talking."

"One of the Warfield maids being scolded for getting herself with child without a husband, perhaps?" he suggested.

"No-o-o-o." She gnawed at her lip. "A long time ago, and much anger."

Too much anger, if she still remembered the episode with such disquiet. He took her hand. "Does the memory make you dislike the thought of babies?"

She shrugged. "It was of no importance. Only a passing thought." She tilted her head to one side pensively. "I've never thought of having children, but I should think I will enjoy them, rather like kittens or puppies."

"Only you would say that." Optimistic that in time she would want children as much as he did, he leaned forward into a kiss. Her lips clung to his, blossom sweet.

She tickled his ribs. Laughing, he set out to discover her ticklish spots. At first they disrobed each other playfully, but soon the kisses and caresses became more urgent until they came together joyously, free of the shadows that had plagued them until now. She was a pagan princess, gloriously naked and at ease in the daisy-spangled grass. A goddess who made his bones melt with passion and fulfillment.

Afterward they lay tangled in the sunshine, both of them gasping for breath. Smoothing back her hair, he said huskily, "I love you, Meriel. Love being with you, love the man I am when I'm with you."

Her eyes closed, but not soon enough to hide her discomfort at his declaration. He wondered, with sudden depression, if she would ever fully return his feelings. Perhaps it was necessary to grow up in normal society, to see the cycles of courtship and marriage, to understand the meaning of human love.

Another thought struck, slow and chilling. Meriel no longer needed him. Marriage had given her the protection required to become the undisputed mistress of Warfield, and it was Warfield she loved, far more than any man or woman.

He drew her close, trying not to think of how he'd promised to leave if she ever asked him to. That wouldn't happen right away. She was fond of him, she trusted him enough to share control of Warfield, and she certainly enjoyed their lovemaking.

But the bonds of love and custom and commitment that held most marriages together were outside her experience. Would the day come when she no longer wished to have him about? Might she lose her temper and send him away in a fit of rage? Or after the first flush of passion between them faded, would she become curious about bedding other men and take lovers? If that happened, he'd leave voluntarily.

Sharply he told himself not to borrow trouble. Certainly Meriel was a passionate mistress who cared for him in her way. He would simply have to take life day by day. If they had children, that would surely forge a deeper bond. And even if she sent him away in a fit of temper, she could always invite him back.

A cloud drifted across the sun, and he wrapped himself around her. They were not only lovers, but friends.

He would pray that was enough.

Chapter 38

Wrexham and Lucia had returned to Dornleigh. *Hell. From his horseback vantage point on top of a hill overlooking the house, Kyle saw the carriage pull up and his father and sister climb out. He promptly turned his horse and rode in the opposite direction. He'd had a couple of days of almost total peace and quiet since returning home, but he still wasn't ready for company.*

He debated whether he should be the one to break the news that Dominic had stolen the heiress Wrexham had wanted for his heir. No, not when that would mean listening to his father bellowing. Besides, the subject was far too painful.

The rage he'd felt in London had burned out, leaving him exhausted and empty. Sooner or later he'd have to do something—but damned if he knew what.

Kyle managed to avoid his father and sister for a day and a half; Dornleigh was large. But the next evening, after a day long expedition to the nearby hills, he returned to his room and found Lucia sitting in his most comfortable chair, reading a book. She glanced up when he entered. "Too late to run—I've seen you."

He considered bolting—the day he couldn't outrun his little sister, he was in trouble—but there was something very undignified about living like a nervous squirrel in his own home. Warily he entered the room. "I should have locked my door before I left."

Lucia closed her book and set it aside. "You can't hide forever. At least I'm on your side, no matter what."

He tossed his hat across the room. It dropped neatly over the corner of a carved wooden chair. "Does that mean you're consigning Dominic to the nethermost regions?"

"I'm on both of your sides," she said quietly. "I know you better, of course, but Dominic is as much my brother as you."

He bit back a furious comment; his quarrel was with Dominic, not Lucia. Brusquely he said, "Do you know what he did?"

She nodded. "Letters from Dominic arrived today for Papa and me. Papa was told the official version of how the marriage came about. Dom told me the complete story because I'd helped him out, and he thought I deserved the truth." She regarded her brother with furrowed brows. "He mentioned that you appeared just after the wedding, and that you were...quite upset to learn of the marriage so abruptly."

"How very euphemistic of him." Mouth tight, Kyle took brandy from a cabinet. He'd brought the decanter up the night he returned to Dornleigh, knowing it would be convenient to have a source of temporary oblivion close at hand.

He poured himself a generous measure and was putting the top back on the decanter when his sister asked, "Aren't you going to offer me any?"

Startled, he said, "You're too young for brandy."

Her brows arched. "I'm of legal age, and on the verge of marriage. Surely I may be permitted a small amount of spirits."

Silently he splashed a finger's worth into another glass and gave it to her, then sprawled in the other, less comfortable chair. "I hope you haven't dropped by for a long sisterly conversation. I'm not in the mood."

"I've already deduced that." She took a careful sip of her brandy. "Did you know that Papa and I visited Warfield when Dominic was there, pretending to be you?"

Kyle stiffened. "Good God, Wrexham knew about the deception that long ago?"

Lucia shook her head. "You know how vain he is about wearing spectacles. He never realized—Dominic imitates you very well. I knew who he was right away, of course, but Dom explained privately why he was there, and asked me not to reveal his identity." She caught his gaze. "I agreed for *both* your sakes."

Kyle couldn't help wincing when he thought about how Dominic must have felt when his family descended on Warfield. He'd probably been tempted to run for his life.

For the first time, Kyle wondered what had happened in his absence. Obviously more had gone wrong than just Dominic seducing Lady Meriel. Reluctantly curious, he said, "You might as well speak your piece. Obviously you won't go away until you have."

"Very true," she agreed. "You need to know the whole story."

He studied his goblet, admiring the rich refraction of candlelight through brandy. "Did Dominic ask you to pacify me? He should have known it wouldn't work."

"Which is why he didn't ask," she retorted. "Talking to you is my idea, because I hate to think that my brothers may spend the rest of their lives completely estranged."

"Accustom yourself," he said tersely. "If I'm lucky, I won't ever see him again. What he did was...unforgivable."

She made a rude noise. "Why? Because you were so in love with Meriel? A man in love would never have asked his brother to court his bride."

He looked up, his mouth tight. "I had my reasons."

Her voice softened. "I'm sure you did, but your actions were not those of a man besotted with his affianced bride. You'd only met her once yourself, hadn't you? Hardly enough to recognize her, much less fall in love."

"You're obsessed with romance," he said, exasperated. "Not everyone makes a love match, as you're doing. Lady Meriel is mentally damaged, not someone a man could fall in love with. The point of the marriage was to ensure that she would be protected from fortune hunters." Anger swept through him again. "Instead, because of my carelessness, the fortune hunter who seduced her is my own brother." Uncomfortably he recognized that guilt was part of his anger—he had failed in his duty, and an innocent, witless girl had suffered for it.

"You looked at Lady Meriel as a pathetic creature in need of protection," Lucia said austerely. "Dominic looked at her, and saw a beautiful woman worthy of love."

"Is that what he's claiming?" Kyle swallowed his remaining brandy and reached for more. "I hadn't realized what a talent he has for lying."

"Kyle, I met Meriel, and found her quite charming," Lucia said earnestly. "According to her chaperons, she began to improve as soon as Dominic came to Warfield. Apparently she is very nearly normal now, and it's Dominic's doing. Could you have done the same for her?"

Kyle paused in the act of pouring. Recollections of what happened at Kimball House were hazy because of the consuming rage he'd felt at the time. He'd scarcely noticed Lady Meriel. She had never been very real to him, least of all on that day, when all his attention was on his brother—but he suddenly remembered that she had spoken, saying in no uncertain terms that it was Dominic she wanted, not him.

Of course she would say that, since Dominic had seduced her and poisoned her mind against her betrothed. But there was no denying that she had talked, and quite coherently. Everyone had assumed the girl was incapable of that, so she must have changed greatly in the short time since Dominic went to Warfield.

Brandy splashed on his hand, and he realized that he'd forgotten the decanter. Flushing at his clumsiness, he took a large swallow, as if he'd intended to pour so much. "If this was a great love match, why did Dominic rush her to the altar with such obscene haste? If he'd waited until I returned and convinced me that he really cared for the girl, I probably would have been willing to bow out on his behalf."

"Dominic had no choice," Lucia said flatly. "Meriel's uncle had locked her up in a madhouse, and Dom wanted to make sure she wasn't sent back there."

"An asylum?" he said, shocked. "Why would Amworth do that? He told me that a major reason for getting the girl a husband was to keep her *out* of the madhouse."

"It was her other uncle, Lord Grahame." Lucia ran a distracted hand through her dark hair. "I'd better start at the beginning."

Tersely she explained that Amworth had become very ill, spurring first Grahame's early return, then an unpleasant string of events that had ended in Dominic breaking Meriel out of the asylum and rushing her into marriage so that he would have legal control over her person. Kyle frowned as he listened, wondering if the tale was true, or just Dominic playing on his sister's desire to think well of him.

Lucia ended, "Dominic has done his best to resolve this without a scandal. The official story, which is what he wrote to Papa, is that you thought he and Meriel would suit, and sent him in your place because of your generous nature."

Kyle gave a bark of harsh laughter. "He really *is* a good liar."

"His version is better than letting the world know you couldn't be bothered to court your own wife," Lucia said tartly. "Did you genuinely want Meriel, or is it that you still can't stand for Dominic to take one of your toys?"

He stared into his brandy, wondering if there might be some truth to his sister's accusation. "This isn't about competition," he said in a raw voice. "I trusted Dominic, and he betrayed me."

She sighed. "Part of me understands that. Another part thinks that a bizarre set of circumstances forced Dominic into doing something that hurt you terribly, but he didn't have much choice if he was to protect the woman he loved." She cocked her head to one side. "Have you ever been in love, Kyle?"

His goblet stem shattered into tinkling fragments, gashing his palm and splashing brandy across his lap. Swearing, he waved Lucia away when she rose to help. As he wrapped the bleeding hand in a towel, he wondered furiously how Dominic dared speak of love. He'd indulged in casual affairs, never spending ten years faithful to a single woman. He'd never held his beloved as she died in his arms....

With horror, Kyle realized that he was on the verge of breaking down in front of his sister. "Get out, Lucia. *Now.*"

A stubborn Renbourne to the core, instead she approached and laid her hand on his arm. "Kyle, I'm so sorry," she whispered. "I can see how horrible the situation has been for you. But can't you accept that this may have been for the best? Dominic loves Meriel. You didn't, but now you have a chance to find a woman you can love."

He jerked away, terrified that he might strike her. "Lucia, you haven't the remotest damned idea what you're talking about," he said raggedly.

"I don't know what it's like to feel betrayed by my twin brother," she said quietly, "but I do know something of love. Because I love Robin, and I love Dominic, and I love you."

He swung away, praying she would leave. After a long moment, her steps moved toward the door, but she paused for a last word. "Dominic and Meriel are holding a community wedding feast on Midsummer Eve. Papa and I are leaving for Warfield tomorrow morning. If you can bring yourself to forgive Dominic, I'm sure you would be welcome, too."

He shook his head, denying her and his brother and the whole hellacious world, where neither love nor trust nor honor endured.

After his sister left, he locked the door, then fell shaking onto his bed, his blood-drenched hand curled against his chest. He should ring for Morrison, who had caught up with him the day after his return to Dornleigh. Though the valet had been unable to prevent the disaster at Warfield, he was quite adept at bandages. But Kyle could not bear the presence of another human, even one as self-effacing as Morrison.

In a dim corner of his churning mind, he realized how much of his fury at Dominic was really rage against the heavens because of Constancia's death. He'd returned from Cádiz clinging to the idea of Lady Meriel, welcoming the fact that she was weak and needy because that would give him something to think about besides his grief.

It had never once occurred to him that she might be capable of recovering, or that she could be a real wife. He didn't *want* a real wife—he'd had one, even if the actual marriage had lasted only for hours. Meriel was infinitely better off with a man who had the patience and understanding to bring her into normal life.

Someone like Dominic, who had always been a healer of injured beasts and unhappy humans.

Would he really have waived his claim on Lady Meriel for Dominic's sake? He wasn't sure—he'd needed the idea of her too much. Without Constancia or Lady Meriel Grahame, who was Kyle? What was the point of his existence? *What was the bloody bedamned point?*

In the midst of anguish, a thread of peace formed, as if Constancia had just entered the room. She had always radiated serenity. He could almost see her lying beside him, her dark eyes warm and profoundly wise.

Fragments of the conversations they'd had on the journey to Spain began tumbling through his mind. *"I would give every valuable I ever possessed for the chance to tell her how much I loved her."* She had wanted him to reconcile with his brother, to avoid the guilt that had plagued her after the savage death of her sister. If something happened to Dominic now, when their relationship was strained to the breaking point, would Kyle be left with guilt for the anger between them?

Damnably, he would.

"Do you envy his freedom? Despise him for not using it the same way you would?" He'd rejected Constancia's words at the time, but now he wondered. Dominic had never wanted to travel to distant places, had never burned with curiosity about the vast, empty spaces of the globe. He'd had the freedom Kyle craved— and had not even noticed because that wasn't what his heart desired.

Instead, Dominic would be an exemplary husband, father, and landowner. He would become a Shropshire magistrate and dispense justice with compassion. Perhaps he should have been the Wrexham heir—yet that honor had fallen to Kyle. The authority of command came naturally to him, and he would never give up his birthright voluntarily, even though that birthright included the responsibility that tied him to England.

Would Kyle and Dominic have stayed friends if the birth order had been reversed? So many of their battles were caused when Kyle tried to impose his idea of the best course on his brother, and Dominic stubbornly refused, even if doing so was cutting off his nose to spite his face.

Would Dominic have been as dictatorial if he'd been the elder? Hard to say—but Kyle would have been equally stubborn if his brother had tried to issue orders.

But Dominic had not been the elder, and over time, an unholy mixture of competition and protectiveness, domination and rebellion, had eroded the bonds forged in their childhood. Kyle now saw with bitter clarity how much of the blame for destroying their relationship belonged to him. He had been the one who had attempted to dominate his brother from pride and anger—and most of all, from a genuine love that had expressed itself badly.

Still, not all the blame was on his side. Despite Lucia's eloquent defense, Kyle suspected that Dominic's motives had been less than pure when he'd rushed Lady Meriel to the altar. Surely there had been a way to protect the girl short of a preemptive marriage. Instead, Dominic had chosen a path guaranteed to hurt and enrage his brother.

With that between them, could they ever be friends again? He doubted it—though perhaps he owed it to himself and Dominic and Constancia to at least try.

He opened his eyes and gazed sightlessly at the ceiling, hearing the last words Constancia had spoken to him. *"For my sake—go forth and live!"*

He wanted to honor her request. But how?

Chapter 39

"Your tenants know how to have a good time," Lord Wrexham said approvingly. Beneath a setting sun, the wedding celebration was in full swing at the base of Castle Hill, with children's games, constant dancing, tables full of food, kegs of drinkables, and quarters of beef being whittled away as they roasted over open fires.

"They do indeed, sir." Dominic, who was sitting on a bench beside his father at the gentry table, was still amazed that the earl had come, and in such an amiable mood. "I think the tenants are pleased to be able to enter Warfield Park and meet their mistress after so many years of rumors." It made them feel safe to know that she was sane and well—and of course, everyone enjoyed a grand party. As a special treat, Jena Ames had spent an hour painting small mehndi designs on the hands and faces of children and excited young girls, and a few brave matrons. East met West, to the approval of all.

His father's gaze went to Meriel, who sat at the other end of the table with Lucia and Jena, who had run out of henna and retired. "You seem to have taught your bride some manners."

"Her manners were always excellent," Dominic said dryly. "It was her self-control that was sometimes lacking." Luckily, his father knew better than to try to pinch his new daughter-in-law's chin again. Meriel was learning to play the gracious lady, but there were distinct limits to her tolerance.

After swallowing his last bite of roast beef, Dominic succumbed to curiosity. "I'm very glad that you and Lucia are here, sir, but to be honest, I'm surprised. I'd thought you would not approve of my marriage when there had been an unofficial betrothal between Maxwell and Lady Meriel."

"I had some doubts about Maxwell marrying Lady Meriel, but the original understanding twenty years ago had involved those two." His father tipped his tankard back to finish his ale. "Besides, I hardly thought I could propose you as a prospective groom when you've disagreed with everything I've ever suggested."

Dominic flushed. "Have I been that bad?"

His father snorted. "Worse. The stubbornest son any father was ever cursed with."

Dominic opened his mouth to protest, then closed it again. He *had* been stubborn, and rebellious as well. Granted, his father's manner was often heavy-handed, but he had not been unreasonable when it mattered most. "I'm sorry if I've caused you grief."

"All children do. Parents and children were put on earth to give each other grief. You were my punishment for how I behaved to my own father." Wrexham's eyes gleamed. "And I'll have my revenge when you have children of your own."

Dominic laughed. "Surely there is more to being a parent than grief."

"Of course there is," his father said gruffly. "Children are the future. What other point is there to life?"

Dominic was startled to hear the emotion in his father's voice. Underneath the habitual brusqueness, apparently his father really did love his children. Dominic had always suspected that the relationship consisted entirely of habit and the need for heirs.

Wrexham frowned. "I know there's been strain between you and your brother, and I suppose this will make things worse." His gaze went to Meriel again. "But I'm glad to see you so well settled in life. You and your bride seem to suit each other, and her fortune is allied to the Renbournes, which is what I wanted. Lucia could have married better, but she and young Justice will do nicely, too. If your brother will find himself a proper wife, the family is in sound shape for another generation."

Once Dominic would have been irritated by his father's mercenary comments. Now that he was a married man, he was surprised to view things differently. When and if he had children, he would be equally concerned to see them well settled, though he was enough of a romantic to weigh the emotional side of marriage more heavily than the financial side.

In fairness, he had to admit that his father had reason to take finances seriously. Having inherited a pile of debts and a run-down estate, Wrexham had worked hard for years to rebuild the family fortunes. It wasn't surprising that money and property played an important role in his calculations for his children.

With wonder, Dominic foresaw a future where he and his father would get along tolerably well, because at heart they shared similar values. Family mattered. The land mattered. Duty mattered. And if his father sometimes irritated him—well, no doubt Dominic could be rather irritating himself. But they would understand each other, and be friends.

Of course he couldn't say anything so sentimental aloud, so he merely offered, "Shall I get you more ale, sir?"

Wrexham shook his head wistfully. "Any more and my gout will lay me out for the next three days."

"A dance, my lord?" A blushing village girl appeared in front of Dominic. She had the air of someone whose friends had egged her into doing something outrageous, and a dark henna flower drying on her right cheek.

"I'm not a lord, but I'd be delighted," he said after a glance at Meriel, who smiled and waved him off. Dominic had been concerned that she would be overwhelmed by the crowd, but her tenants had been shyly respectful, albeit burning with curiosity about the mad Lady Meriel who had been their unseen mistress for so many years.

He followed the girl into the squares forming for a country dance. He and Meriel had led off the dancing, and enjoyed themselves thoroughly. So far she had showed no signs of tiring of his presence. Quite the contrary.

The fiddler began to play, and people swung into the figures of the dance. Dominic laughed at the startled expression of a middle-aged woman whom he twirled around; she hadn't realized that the new lord of the manor was in the same set. But her shock was followed by a toothy smile. The locals seemed to have accepted him wholeheartedly. He'd never be the distant sort of master his father was.

In the adjoining square, Lucia was dancing with face flushed and ribbons flying, partnered by young Jem Brown, the former poacher, who looked well fed and content. The same set contained John Kerr. The steward knew his own worth, but he'd still been relieved by Dominic's reassurance that his services were needed and valued.

Soon dusk would be advanced enough to set the huge bonfire ablaze. Dominic privately thought there was something rather pagan about a bonfire on Midsummer Eve, but that was all right. This was a very pagan sort of celebration.

Meriel tapped her foot to the music as she watched Dominic dance with the girl. He was so good with people, kind but also a natural leader. Every tenant and villager in Warfield already adored him, and who could blame them? Luckily, he didn't expect her to be a belle of the ball, even at her own marriage feast. He understood.

Deciding she needed to stretch her legs, she slid from the bench and began to circle the festivities. This was the longest day of the year, but finally the sun was sinking toward the horizon, and the slanting rays were turning the fields and the old castle above to molten gold. Her home had never been more lovely, or more loved.

"Milady." Kamal fell into step beside her, looking majestic in his neatly coiled turban and well-cut tunic.

She smiled up at him. "At the spring equinox, who would have imagined such a scene at the summer solstice?"

"No one." He glanced over the crowd toward the gentry table. Lord and Lady Amworth were there, along with two of their children, who were about Meriel's age. The cousins were amiable, and the countess kept a close eye on her husband to ensure that he didn't overexert himself. Mrs. Rector and

Mrs. Marks were chatting with the general and Jena Ames, and even Lord Grahame was speaking politely to the parish vicar.

"There has been much change, and will be more." Kamal regarded her seriously. "The time has come for me to leave Warfield, milady."

"Oh, no!" She stopped in her tracks, dismayed. "Are you going home to India?"

"England is my home now, but I am no longer needed at Warfield. You have a husband to look after you."

"That doesn't mean I don't still need you," she whispered, a lump in her throat.

"I shan't go far," Kamal said reassuringly. "General Ames is getting along in years, and wishes help in managing Holliwell Grange. Though the house is not so grand as Warfield, the estate is nearly as large. He has asked me to become his steward."

"I see." Meriel suddenly understood. "Will you and Jena be happy, Kamal?"

He stared, more surprised than she'd ever seen him. "How did you know?"

She smiled blandly. "I have my ways."

He laughed. "I should have known you would realize. Yes, milady, Jena and I will be happy. We have known each other in other lifetimes, I think." He resumed walking, his expression pensive. "Even as a child, I felt that I was not properly rooted in my homeland. When the time was right, I came to England to watch over you. Now that you are well, it is time to take the next step on my path."

Meriel realized that General Ames had to know about the relationship. By hiring Kamal, he was giving tacit approval. And well he should—he could look the world over and not find a more honorable man for Jena. "I'm glad you won't be far away."

"I'll always be near if you need me, little flower," he said softly.

She blinked back tears. It was hard to describe exactly what the relationship was between them—there were elements of father, big brother, and friend. Whatever the definition, his kindness and love had kept her sane. "How did we first meet? You've been so much a part of my life that I can't even remember."

"Perhaps it is for the best if you don't recall."

She stared at him. "That statement begs questions."

"I don't mean to be mysterious." His expression was troubled. "If you feel the need to know, I shall tell you."

She did want to know, but not tonight. Something was tugging at the back of her mind. Her memories of India were a chaotic jumble of terror and intense sensations and sudden, startling beauty. She had always tried not to think of the past, but perhaps it was time she did.

The dance had ended, and Dominic was holding a small blond, somewhere in the vicinity of four years old. Meriel felt a squeeze on her heart at the sight. He would make a wonderful father—and his children would be *her* children. For the first time, she experienced the primal desire to have a baby, but not just any child. His.

She glanced away, not wanting to allow her emotions to get out of hand in public. Idly she noticed a horseman cantering toward the gathering from the direction of the house. She shaded her eyes and tried to see, wondering who was coming so late. She'd thought that any guest who would have a horse was already here.

A travel-stained young man, well dressed. Handsome but stern, looking rather like Dominic, but with a darker, more restless light...

She gasped. Alerted by some instinct, Dominic glanced up and saw the horseman. For an instant he was very still. Then he gently handed the little girl back to her mother and began walking through the crowd toward the newcomer.

Kamal said sharply, "Is something wrong?"

"Not if I can help it!" Meriel flung over her shoulder as she raced off, determined to be present when Dominic and his twin brother met again.

Dominic tried to read Kyle's expression but could see nothing beyond brittle self-control—and a swift glimpse of a pocket pistol as his brother swung off his horse. He stiffened as an image of Kyle pulling out the gun and coolly taking aim seared across his mind. Reminding himself that it was normal to carry a weapon when traveling alone, he said in a neutral voice, "I didn't expect to see you here."

Before his brother could reply, Meriel materialized, panting and looking like a furious angel. "Lord Maxwell," she said flatly. "If you are here to insult my husband again, I will personally scratch your eyes out."

"You have a fierce defender." Kyle studied his sister-in-law intently, then gave a slight bow. "You may sheathe your claws, Lady Meriel. I did not come here to fight."

"Then why did you come?" Dominic's gaze went to where his brother's coat concealed the pistol. "To administer justice?"

Kyle flushed, understanding immediately. "Of course not. I just came...to talk. Will you walk with me?" He glanced at Meriel and Kamal, who had appeared at a more leisurely pace. "Alone."

Though Meriel looked mutinous, Kamal said, "Of course." After collecting the horse's reins, he deftly removed Meriel.

Dominic fell into step beside his brother, who set a course away from the gathering. Silently they followed along a hedgerow, until Kyle said, "Lucia cornered me and explained at some length your version of events. Was it true?"

Dominic studied his brother's profile, which could have been carved from granite. "I shouldn't think that she made anything up."

Kyle was silent for another dozen steps before asking, "Can you honestly say that when you married Meriel, it wasn't at least partly from a desire to score over me?"

Hell. What was the right answer to a question like that?

When in doubt, tell the truth. Ruthlessly Dominic dissected the motives behind what had been an excruciating decision before replying, "I don't think so. Mostly I was terrified that if Lord Grahame found Meriel, he'd take her back to the asylum. When Kamal and I went to Bladenham, she was tied to a chair in a straitjacket, like a wild beast. I couldn't allow that to happen again."

Kyle gave him a shocked glance. "My God, her uncle permitted that?"

"He thought he was giving her the best available treatment." Dominic hesitated, then continued haltingly, "While most of my concern was for her, if I'm going to be completely honest I have to admit that I also wanted to make her *mine*—to bind her in marriage so that no one could take her away from me."

"So your love for the lady was greater than your loyalty to me," Kyle said coolly.

Dominic swore to himself. They'd never had a discussion that cut so close to the core of their conflicts, and now he saw why. This level of honesty was devilishly uncomfortable. "I swear by all that's holy that having to hurt you in order to protect Meriel was the most damnably difficult thing I've ever done. If I hadn't truly feared that she might end up in

435

the madhouse, I would have waited for you to return so we could have settled the question face-to-face."

His brother sighed, some of the tension fading. "I'm glad to hear that. I was afraid you had seized on the opportunity to pay me back for being born first."

"I have never wanted to harm you, even when things were most strained between us," Dominic said quietly. "Believe that if nothing else."

"I do believe it, because I've always felt the same." Kyle picked an ox-eye daisy from the hedgerow, rolling the stem between his fingers. "That was why it was so upsetting to think that the…the underlying trust had been violated."

So that feeling of trust had not been just on Dominic's side. "In this case, Meriel had to come first—and I hope I never have to make such a decision again."

"I suppose I faced a similar decision and didn't choose Meriel, so perhaps it's only fair that I lost her," Kyle said pensively. "She has been completely transformed since the first time we met. She looks very pretty, and doesn't seem the least bit witless. The credit for that goes to you, I gather."

"She was never witless, and has done as much for me as I have done for her." Dominic stopped himself from trying to explain why she entranced him. Another time, perhaps. At the moment, it was more important to seize this chance to clear the thickets of misunderstanding that had separated him and his brother for so long.

He moistened dry lips before asking the vital question. "For years, I've hoped that someday we could be friends again. Is that possible?"

His brother halted and turned to meet his gaze. In Kyle's eyes were pain, wariness, and a yearning to connect that was as strong as Dominic's. "I...I don't know. We've been at cross-purposes for so long."

Realizing that his brother needed a reason to believe, Dominic said, "We're not in competition any more, Kyle, if we ever were. Maybe now it will be possible to simply relax and accept each other's differences."

Kyle gave a swift smile that reminded Dominic of when they had been boys and closeness had been as instinctive as breathing. "God knows that it's worth trying."

"Shall we shake on it?" Dominic took his brother's hand, then hastily dropped it when Kyle winced. Glancing down, he saw a stained bandage across his brother's palm. It must have hurt to hold reins during a long ride. "What happened?"

"Cut glass. Nothing important." Kyle closed his hand over the bandage. He'd always preferred to conceal weakness, which made it all the more remarkable that he had chosen to try to bridge the gap between them.

But perhaps it wasn't so remarkable, because Kyle had changed over the last weeks. Dominic tried to define the difference, and decided that his brother looked as if he'd been forged in a fire by God's own blacksmith. Petty concerns had been burned away, leaving pure steel. In fact, they had both changed profoundly in these last weeks, though for different reasons and in different ways.

Maybe now they were finally mature enough to avoid the tension and conflicts of the past. Dominic asked, "What took you out of the country so that you couldn't come to Warfield yourself?"

Kyle raised his brows. "How did you know I was out of the country?"

"I was receiving some rather strong messages from you. Very unhappy ones."

Kyle's face tightened. "You were always good at that." After a long silence, he said in a voice saturated with pain, "I was...taking the woman I loved to Spain to die."

"Damnation." Dominic caught his breath, recognizing that this explained everything—Kyle's outrageous bribe to persuade Dominic to take his place, the anguish that had radiated from him on his journey, the volatile, desperate anger that had exploded against Dominic at Kimball House. "I'm sorry."

He imagined how he'd feel if something happened to Meriel, and his belly clenched. After seeking a way to give comfort and finding none, he put his hand on his brother's shoulder and repeated, "I'm so sorry."

He felt a flicker of response, and knew that Kyle understood what Dominic was unable to put into words. Clearly his brother could not bear to say more about a wound that was still so raw—but then, what more needed to be said? A single terse sentence contained a whole tragedy.

Dominic took a deep breath. Kyle had revealed his own vulnerability, and Dominic could do no less. He yearned to tell his brother the story of Waterloo—the pain and fear and craziness. Enough time had passed that he could speak clearly of the experience that had changed his life, and left him adrift for so many years.

Talk was the best way to build bridges, and they had a lot of building to do.

Chapter 40

Impatiently Meriel watched in the direction where Dominic and his brother had vanished. She half expected them to beat each other to a bloody pulp, so it was a great relief when they finally reappeared. Obviously they had resolved their differences—she could see it in the relaxed way they moved, and in the way Dominic laughed and Lord Maxwell clapped him on the back. They both looked younger and much happier. She might actually come to like Maxwell, if he didn't trouble Dominic again.

As Maxwell paused at the spit to collect a plate of sliced beef from the cook, Dominic appeared beside Meriel, putting an arm around her waist for a surreptitious squeeze. "You're holding up well," he said cheerfully. "Not much longer."

"Good. I shall be ready to retire." Meriel glanced up at him through her lashes. "I'm glad you and your brother have made your peace."

"So am I. We talked out almost twenty years' worth of misunderstandings." His arm tightened around her. "Oddly enough, I think maybe it's for the best that we went our separate ways for so long. We've each grown in our own fashion, and now we can just accept each other as we are. He doesn't have to dominate, and I don't need to rebel."

Meriel doubted that she would ever understand the subtleties of being a twin, but no matter. Dominic was happy, and that was enough.

Finally it was growing dark, and everyone in the parish had apparently eaten enough, drunk enough, and danced enough. The last event was the bonfire. It was heralded when Lord Grahame crossed to the head-high pile of wood and boomed, "It's time to light the Midsummer fire, and may it blaze through the shortest night of the year in honor of the marriage of Dominic and Lady Meriel!"

Her uncle was carrying a massive, brass-headed cane, and he waved it in the air for emphasis. He claimed to have twisted his ankle, though Meriel suspected that he'd been so angry when she showed up with Dominic and the Ameses that he'd gone upstairs and kicked the wardrobe, bruising his foot. He'd behaved impeccably ever since, so she supposed he was entitled to one fit of temper.

As the crowd gathered, Dominic murmured, "Wait here a moment. I want to escort Kyle over to my father and sister, so that they can see we're civil again."

Meriel nodded, glad to avoid the family reunion. It would take time for Dominic to make his way back to her, but she was comfortable even without him by her side. These were her people, and she could feel their goodwill.

Kerr, the steward, struck a spark to ignite Lord Grahame's torch. Her uncle turned toward her and called, "Meriel, will you set the Midsummer fire?"

She repressed a shiver. Bonfires had never appealed to her—they reminded her too much of how her parents had died. "Please do the honors, Uncle."

Grahame swung around and hurled his torch into the waiting wood. Flammable materials had been stuffed into cracks, so the fire caught instantly. As flames shot into the air, screams of excitement rose from the crowd.

Meriel froze, feeling as if she had been clubbed. The arch of her uncle's body as he flung the torch, the flames, the screams...Terror lanced through her, swift and violent as lightning.

Consumed by panic, she whirled and cut through the crowd, flying toward the safety of the night. She emerged by the path that ran up Castle Hill, so she darted into it, stumbling over stones and roots as she climbed toward the ruins.

She reached the castle's inner bailey before a stitch in her side forced her to stop. Gasping for breath, she folded onto the grass and pressed her hand to her side as she tried to make sense of the fear coursing through her. Images from her nightmares churned through her mind—scenes of fire and fear and evil, and the dark man who threw the first torch. Screams of menace, cries of desperation from those trapped in the flames.

And...Kamal? He was there, too, younger, less lined, but unmistakable.

Far below, she could see the blazing fire and the people gathered around it, heedless of her private torment. She wrapped her arms around herself, shivering, and grimly forced herself to seek the truth buried in her nightmare.

Wrexham and Lucia were delighted to see Kyle, especially since he and Dominic were obviously on easy terms again. Leaving his brother with the rest of the family, Dominic headed back to Meriel. He was still some distance away when he saw her suddenly dart from the bonfire. He frowned, wondering if the press of people had finally become too much for her. Concerned, he worked his way through the laughing villagers. It was time to take his wife home.

Traces of the long twilight lingered in the sky, and an orange gibbous moon cast light as well. Even so, he had to pick his steps cautiously as he followed her up Castle Hill. Knowing the ground so well, Meriel had probably gone this way at full speed. At least she wore a light-colored dress, so he should be able to find her in the dark.

He was beginning to wonder if she might have left the path and returned to the house when he entered the old castle precinct, and saw a ghostly figure crumpled on the ground. Hastening to her, he asked, "Meriel, is something wrong?"

She looked up at him, her face deathly pale in the moonlight. He knelt and put his arms around her. "What happened?"

Trembling violently, she buried her face against him, radiating fear. Wondering what could cause such a reaction, he asked, "Were you assaulted?"

"N-no." Her voice was barely audible. "I was...remembering."

A chill ran through him as he realized what must be in her mind. "Did the bonfire and the shouting remind you of the night your parents died?"

Instead of answering, she lurched to her feet and crossed to the ancient stone steps that ran up to the parapet. Alarmed, Dominic followed, staying within an arm's length. When she went to the battlements, he almost dragged her back.

Bracing her hands on the stone, she stared starkly into the darkness. "The moon was like tonight's. I was on a balcony like this, looking out at the stars and afraid my nurse would come and take me back to bed. The main section of the palace was there." She gestured to the right. "Alwari wasn't heavily fortified, for it was not the chief royal residence. The maharajah's capital city was two days farther north, but he'd given my father permission to stay at Alwari to honor the British emissary."

Quietly he asked, "Did you see the raiders attack?"

Her posture was rigid, and he guessed that she was seeing India rather than the quiet Shropshire night. "They galloped in like thunder, shouting and waving torches. There were dozens and dozens—an army of savages, firing guns and waving spears. They overwhelmed my father's escort, which was small because we were supposed to be in safe territory. Our people were caught completely off guard."

She took a ragged breath. "One raider was dressed all in black, his face covered except for his eyes. He was not the leader, but he threw the first torch. It was the dry season, and the roof caught fire and blazed up like tinder. The dark man was mad, I think, perhaps sworn to destroy the foreigners, for he rode his screaming horse right into the palace. I did not see him come out again."

She was shivering. He put his arm around her shoulders, wanting to anchor her to the present. "So you saw it all happen."

She pulled at her braid, her fingers kneading

frantically. "As people fled the fire, they were cut down by swords and spears. Every one of them. There was a sweet old man who had brought me sherbet. His...his head was cut off, and one of the raiders used the butt of his spear to knock it across the courtyard."

"Dear God," he whispered. No wonder she hadn't wanted to remember this slaughter. What a horror for a child. For anyone. "Did you see your parents?"'

She shook her head. "Their rooms were right under where the roof caught fire. I...I hope they died swiftly from the smoke."

That would have been a mercy, if true. "How the devil did you escape?"

"I was terrified of the fire, but I was also too frightened to jump. The courtyard was so far down, and filled with those brutes. I huddled into a ball, shrieking, afraid I'd be spitted like a pig on someone's spear," she said haltingly. "Then my nurse, Hiral, staggered up behind me. She...her robe was on fire. She shouted into the night, and a rider just below the balcony reined in his horse and looked up.

"It was the strangest thing. They stared at each other for what seemed like forever. I...I think the man was shocked to see a burning woman and a child there." Meriel began to weep. "Hiral screamed something that made the hair on my head stand up. Then...then she picked me up and threw me over the railing."

"Jesus Christ." He caught her to him, shaking as badly as she at the vivid horror she had described. "The raider caught you?"

445

"I...I think he must have," she whispered into his shoulder. "I was falling, and then I slammed to a halt. The next I remember is being carried across a horse, a man's hand on my back, feeling as if my bones would jolt from my skin."

He enfolded her, desperately wishing he could take her pain away. "You're safe now, love, you're safe. It's all over."

"But it isn't," she whispered. *"It isn't."*

Ravenous from his long ride, Kyle was attacking the excellent food when Lucia settled next to him in a flurry of skirts. "Have you and Dominic truly settled your differences, or were you just pretending for the sake of Papa and me?"

He washed down a mouthful of beef and bread. "We really did, Lucia. You deserve the credit for making me listen when I didn't want to."

She exhaled with relief. "I'm so glad. Do you think this will last?"

"Yes. We both want peace, and there no longer seems anything to fight about." Beyond that, Kyle felt as if Constancia's death had changed him in some fundamental manner, freeing him in ways he did not yet fully understand.

"The two of you could not have presented me with a better wedding gift." Smiling, Lucia gave him a quick hug, then went to join the revelers surrounding the bonfire.

Kyle was about to carve off another piece

of beef when he paused, knife in the air. Something was wrong, and it concerned Dominic. Danger? A chill went through him. Uneasily he got to his feet and scanned the crowd, but even when he climbed on the bench for a better view, he couldn't find Dominic.

When was the last time he'd seen him? Vaguely he remembered Lady Meriel leaving the crowd, followed shortly thereafter by Dominic. Kyle had guessed that the newlyweds intended a private celebration. There could be no danger in that, not inside a walled private park.

Could someone else have gone off that way? Perhaps a thief had entered Warfield along with the villagers, and waited to catch one of the gentry alone for a robbery.

Nonsense. His imagination was running riot. He climbed down from the bench and reached for his tankard, then halted. His uneasiness was growing stronger. There weren't likely to be any criminals nearby, but Dominic and Meriel had been heading toward the old castle, a place that must have dangerous crumbling stones.

Abandoning his dinner, he skirted the crowd and went to the foot of the path that ran up to the castle. He might embarrass them all by finding Dominic and Meriel in an intimate moment, but he could not ignore the hum of warning in the back of his mind.

He had just reached the path when a tall, dark shape materialized beside him. It was

Kamal. The Indian asked, "Is something amiss, my lord?"

Kyle shrugged, a little embarrassed. "It's probably foolish, but I've been feeling some concern for my brother."

"Oddly, I have also felt concern for Lady Meriel. Perhaps we should investigate together." Despite the softness of Kamal's voice, it was not a request.

As they headed up the hill, Kyle decided that perhaps an ally might be useful.

Dominic looked down at Meriel, trying to read her expression in near-darkness. "What do you mean, it isn't over?"

She swallowed. "The argument I remembered about babies? It was between my father and my uncle. I overheard them at Cambay a few days before we left the cantonment. I...I think my father was breaking the news that my mother had conceived again, and of course if she had a boy, his brother would no longer be the heir."

Dominic sucked in his breath. "And Grahame was angry, even though he had to have known it was a possibility."

Meriel rubbed her temple with stiff fingers. "I wasn't born until my parents had been married for years. More years had passed, so another child must have been a great shock to my uncle. He exploded, shouting that he had borrowed money on his expectations, and what would he do now?

"My father said he'd settle the debts this once

448

but not again, so my uncle must learn to live within his income. My uncle swore, then apologized, saying he'd be more careful, since he was no longer sure of inheriting the earldom. But he was so *furious*. I...I keep wondering if he might have had something to do with the massacre."

Dominic was about to say that was unlikely when a cold voice cut through the night. "So you remembered. I was afraid of that as soon as you started talking again."

A dark form took shape and weight in the night as Grahame mounted the last of the stone steps. He halted, cane in hand, and regarded Meriel thoughtfully. "I assumed that you died at Alwari. It was quite a shock when you reappeared, but as long as you were mad and mute, I could afford to let you live." Idly he drew the cane through his fingers. "It really would have been much better for you to have stayed mad."

There was death in that cool, casual voice. Instinctively stalling for time, Dominic released Meriel and edged between her and her uncle. "Did you really arrange that raid?"

"I was a liaison to the Maharajah of Kanphar," he said calmly. "Knowing that he had an unofficial bandit army in the hill country, I made a bargain with him. He would send his raiders to Alwari, and I would go along to see that the thing was done properly. The bandits would get the loot, while I guaranteed the maharajah certain concessions in an agreement that was being negotiated with Kanphar."

His teeth showed whitely in the dark. "A satisfactory arrangement for all concerned."

"My God," Dominic said, stunned. "You murdered your own brother and his wife! How many others died at Alwari to satisfy your greed?"

Grahame shrugged. "Perhaps a hundred. Most were Hindus, who believe their fates are preordained. I was merely an instrument of their destiny. I put my own life in the hands of fate by riding into the palace, but destiny was with me. I rode straight through and out the other side, and away to safety." He smiled a little. "Of course I'd visited Alwari and knew the palace. Still, if the gods had wished to strike me down for impiety, they could have done it. They chose to let me live."

With a quick twist, he unscrewed the head of the cane. The damnable device divided into two weapons, one a glittering sword stick and the other a short, heavy brass club.

Behind Dominic, Meriel hissed like a wildcat. Guessing that she was on the verge of assaulting her uncle, Dominic caught her wrist, immobilizing her. Better for her to run. Knowing the ruins, with a head start she should be able to escape.

He moved a step toward Grahame. "I assume you intend to kill us both or you wouldn't have said so much, but surely two murders will be a bit conspicuous."

"Not at all. Despite Meriel's little spell of apparent normalcy, everyone knows she's mad. So tragic that she killed herself on the night of her wedding celebration. A jump from the castle wall into the river, her husband gallantly losing his life in an attempt to save her." The older man smiled again, cold as an executioner. "So thoughtful of you to come up here. I had been toying with other schemes—poison, suicide with her father's dueling pistols, perhaps a fall—but they were more complicated. Riskier. This is far better. With you dying together, I shall inherit the hundred thousand pounds that my brother left Meriel. A pity that the estate will go back to Amworth's family, but one can't have everything."

Damnation, Grahame's plan just might work, with no one suspecting foul play. Even stab wounds would go unnoticed on bodies that spent a day or two in the river. Knowing there would be no better chance, Dominic yelled, "Run, Meriel!"

Shoving her behind him, he dived low at the older man, hoping to bring him down. In a hand-to-hand fight, he'd have a good chance, and Meriel could escape.

But Grahame was prepared. Sidestepping swiftly, he slammed the brass club into Dominic's skull. After an instant of shattering pain, the world vanished into blackness.

Chapter 41

Meriel screamed as Dominic crumpled to the walkway, still as death. Why did the

451

fool man have to go after her uncle? They both might have escaped if he hadn't tried to be so damnably noble!

Rigid with panic, she dropped on her knees beside her husband. Dear God, how could she survive without him?

Though a trickle of blood ran down his temple, he still breathed. She touched his cheek with trembling fingers. He wasn't dead, not yet.

But neither of them would see the dawn if Grahame had his way. Why had she never realized he was behind the death of her parents, and so many others? Pieces of the truth had been in her mind, but she had refused to look, preferring her safe, private world of apparent madness, where there were no unbearable memories or murderous uncles.

Consumed by rage, she looked up at Grahame, who stood a yard away and watched her with lightless eyes. "You filthy, hell-born *bastard*!"

"Such language, my dear. You really are an uncivilized little creature." He raised the club. "I'd prefer to use this, since any bruises on your corpse will appear to have been caused by your fall, but I'll spit you if that's what you prefer." He made a grand sweep with the sword stick. "After all, you're my only niece, so I'll extend that courtesy."

She snapped, "If there is madness in this family, it is yours."

"Mad? Not at all. Merely supremely pragmatic." He dropped the sword stick behind him and stepped toward her, the brass club poised.

He expected her to wait weakly for her doom. Gauging her moment, Meriel sprang like a cat as he struck, dodging under the blow.

The club grazed her right arm with numbing intensity, but caused no major damage and left her uncle off balance. She darted past on the narrow edge of walkway between Grahame and the drop to the castle bailey. Scooping up the sword stick, she whirled, the blade secure in both hands. "You thought Dominic was the dangerous one, but you were wrong," she said with lethal intensity. "For hurting him, you will die."

He blinked, startled by the swift turn of events. Then he laughed. "You think that a child like you can injure a trained soldier?" He lunged, seeking to disarm her.

As he caught her shoulder, she stabbed underneath his grasping arms. The blade slashed along his ribs, ripping through his shirt. Warm blood splashed on her as she wrenched free of his grip and retreated.

"You little *bitch*!" Grahame touched the wound, then looked at the dark stain on his fingers with disbelief. "For that, your death will be far more painful."

"There will be no deaths here tonight." The deep voice came from Kamal, who was racing up the steps behind Grahame three at a time, a curved dagger in his hand.

As Grahame swore, Meriel said, "Shall we slice him into ribbons, Kamal?"

"No, milady," Kamal said gently. "He is mine. If I had known he was the devil responsible for the massacre at Alwari, I would have killed him long since."

Grahame dropped the club and yanked a double-barreled pistol from under his coat. "A gun is riskier, but you've left me no choice." He cocked the hammer and aimed at Kamal. "No one will hear a gunshot over the shouting at the bonfire."

"Kamal!" Meriel screamed. A sharp, double crack split the night. One pistol shot or two? There was a clatter of metal as a cloud of black powder stung her eyes.

Another voice—Dominic's?—barked, "Meriel, grab his gun!"

No, not Dominic, Maxwell, who had come up the steps behind Kamal. Meriel dropped the sword stick from the walkway and darted forward to snatch the pistol that had spun away from her uncle. The barrels were gouged—Maxwell had shot the gun from Grahame's hand, making the bullet meant for Kamal go astray.

"It's all over, you bastard," Maxwell snapped. "You're outnumbered and out of weapons, and if you've seriously hurt my brother, I will borrow Kamal's knife and help Meriel cut you into small, bloody pieces."

"Three against one aren't very sporting odds," Kamal observed as he moved, soft-footed and implacable, toward Grahame.

"I don't give a damn about sportsmanship at the moment," Maxwell said with menacing coldness, his expression vividly demonstrating how much he differed from his brother. Dominic was the civilized man, Meriel realized. She, like Maxwell, was a bloodthirsty savage beneath the skin. No wonder she hadn't had any desire to marry him—they were too much alike. It was Dominic who owned her soul.

Dizzy with relief that the danger was past, she dropped the pistol and stepped toward her husband, who lay unmoving between her and Grahame. She was uttering a fervent prayer that his injury was not serious when her uncle seized her, sweeping her so high that her feet dangled in the air. "I may die," he snarled, "but not alone!"

He swung her around toward the river and clambered up into an embrasure. She struggled violently, knowing that this area of the wall was a sheer drop, but Grahame was too large, too strong and enraged. He lurched forward, and she felt the horrifying emptiness of the abyss beneath her, saw moonlight glinting on water far, far below.

Then strong arms locked around her legs. For a ghastly moment she was being torn in half. Then she was wrenched from Grahame's grip and dragged back to safety. She crashed to the walkway as her uncle's scream echoed from the ancient castle walls.

Dazed, she realized that Dominic had ripped her free with the weight of his own body, pulling her down on top of him. Ignoring her bruises, she wrapped herself around his warm, familiar form. "You're all right!"

He gave a shaky laugh. "I don't know if I'd go that far—my head is going to ache for the next week—but I think I'll survive."

Weeping, she buried her face against his neck. "I love you, Dominic. Don't you *dare* die before me."

He became very still. "If you love me, Meriel, I may just live forever."

The moment of privacy ended as Maxwell knelt beside them. "You weren't hurt badly, Dom?" Carefully he brushed back his brother's hair, revealing a bloody laceration.

"I blacked out, but I'm better than I have any right to expect." Dominic shakily pushed himself to a sitting position, then got to his feet with his brother's help.

"A good thing it was your head Grahame hit," Maxwell said lightly. "That's too hard to damage."

As Dominic laughed, Meriel glanced at Kamal, who stood by the parapet, gazing down into blackness. "Is there any chance my uncle might survive the fall to the river?"

"None at all," the Indian said pensively. "The wheels of karma grind slow, but they grind exceeding fine."

She suspected that he was taking liberties with several sets of sacred text, but there were more important questions to ask. "Tonight I remembered everything that happened at Alwari. You were there, weren't you, Kamal?"

He turned from the river and regarded her with eyes as deep as eternity. "I was one of the many sons of the Maharajah of Kanphar. Not

456

the heir, but an officer in my father's army. Sometimes I rode with his bandits to assure they did not exceed his wishes and wreak too much havoc." His voice became heavily ironic. "It was a most important, responsible position. Great things were expected of me."

Quietly Meriel moved to stand in front of him. "So we met at the massacre."

Kamal's face twisted. "I knew there was something different that night, for the raiders were joined by a stranger, a fanatic who spoke Urdu like a native and cried out for British blood. Though I disliked our mission, I did my part in the destruction—until I heard a scream. I looked up, and on the balcony above was a burning woman, the most terrifying sight I have ever seen."

"Hiral cursed you, didn't she?" Meriel had picked up enough Hindi to catch the gist of that tormented cry.

He nodded. "She commanded me to save you, on pain of my own soul. Then she dropped you into my arms. You were fragile as a bird, your silver hair flying about you. As I held you, I had a...a revelation about the sacredness of life. For the first time I truly understood the consequences of the violence that had been my path."

An image flashed through her mind: Kamal's horror-struck expression, the light of the burning palace in his eyes as he held her safe. "So you rescued me, and took me to the zenana."

He spread his hands eloquently. "I knew you

would be safe there. Despite my recognition that I could no longer be a warrior, it took me many months to realize that a different life was impossible as long as I was my father's son. Then I heard that you were to be given in marriage to a neighboring prince. I went to my father and suggested that it would be better to return you to the English, who would be most grateful."

Meriel nodded, seeing the rest. "You went to Cambay, and were asked if you would escort Mrs. Madison and me back to England." Her uncle had long since left India, so there had been no one at the fort to recognize that Kamal had been part of the original raid. He had merely been a polite, well-educated Indian who could be trusted to serve well. "You were a prince, and Mrs. Madison thought you a harem guard."

"I was grateful for that—it separated me from my past, and provided a path to penance. But one lifetime will not be enough to atone for my crimes." He regarded her stoically. "I cannot expect you to forgive me my part in the massacre, when I cannot forgive myself."

Tears stinging her eyes, she went into his arms. "Of course I forgive you, for you have been my salvation."

He hugged her for a moment. "Thank you, little flower."

She stepped away from him, feeling that the door had just closed on the first phase of her life. Now she understood what she was, and why.

Maxwell said thoughtfully, "Much as I'd like

to see Grahame's name blackened as it deserves, I suppose it's more discreet to simply allow it to appear that his death was accidental."

Meriel shivered as she thought of the attention that would be drawn by a public revelation of her uncle's crimes. No one would benefit by the resulting scandal. "The less said about that beast, the better."

She turned to Dominic, who enfolded her with warmth and tenderness. Though she had been slow to recognize love, she understood it now, for it blazed in her heart, searing every fiber of being with passion and protection, friendship and bone-deep commitment. "Once you said that you would leave Warfield if I asked you to. If I'm ever mad enough to ask—don't go."

He laughed and kissed her ear. "Don't worry, my love. I'm not sure I would be gentleman enough to keep my word about that."

She burrowed against him, feeling the strong beat of his heart beneath her ear. "You don't have to be a gentleman, as long as you never, ever leave me."

Epilogue

Efficient as always, Lady Lucia Renbourne had managed to pick a perfect September day for her wedding. Her marriage was in the parish church at Dornleigh so longtime neighbors could attend.

The ceremony went smoothly, except when the nervous groom dropped the ring, which rolled halfway across the church's stone floor before being retrieved by the groomsman. Dominic sympathized entirely—he'd been a bundle of nerves even though there'd been a much smaller audience when he and Meriel married.

The ceremony ended in a radiant kiss, after which the guests poured into the churchyard to await the bride and groom. Dominic made sure that Meriel was firmly attached to his arm. Though she was much more relaxed in crowds than she had been, it was altogether too easy to misplace someone her size.

As children rushed happily about waving sticks with ribbons rippling from the end, people chatted and small baskets of rose petals were distributed for later use. Growing restless, Meriel surveyed the well-planted churchyard. "I'll be right back."

As she darted off, Dominic noted with a grin that even though her pale green gown was impeccable and her hair was elegantly coiled beneath a flowered bonnet, she'd shed her shoes in favor of grass beneath her feet. Beside him, Kyle's voice said thoughtfully, "I'm glad to see that she isn't yet fully civilized."

"I think there's no danger of that," Dominic said with a private smile as he thought of the previous night. There was much to be said for marrying a passionate pagan.

He turned to his brother. They'd not had a chance to talk privately since Dominic and Meriel had arrived at Dornleigh the day before, but clearly Kyle was far more relaxed than the last time they'd seen each other, at Warfield. Then he had been stretched to the snapping point from the loss of the woman he loved, and from his feelings of betrayal. Now he looked...balanced. Comfortable with himself in a way that Dominic hadn't seen since they were boys.

Kyle remarked, "Have you talked to Wrexham yet? Since Meriel has no close male relatives on the Grahame side, the old boy is plotting to get the title settled on you and her." He grinned. "So you can finally be an earl."

"Good God," Dominic said blankly.

"Would you enjoy being the next Lord Grahame?"

Dominic hesitated. "A title doesn't really seem that important." The real treasure was his wife, not her family earldom. "I'll ask Meriel how she feels about it."

Kyle's expression sobered. "I'm going to leave England, Dominic. I don't know when I'll be back." He nodded toward the church. "I stayed long enough for Lucia's wedding, but tomorrow I'm off."

"Damnation," Dominic said involuntarily. He bit back the childish desire to try to change his brother's mind. Kyle deserved the chance to find his own kind of happiness. "I...we'll miss you."

"And I'll miss you," his brother said quietly. "It's ironic to do this just when you and I have finally made our peace. But if I don't go now, I never will."

461

"What does Wrexham have to say about this?"

"I'll tell him tonight. He won't be happy, but he has you and Meriel to take care of the succession if something happens to me." Kyle hesitated, searching for words. "I've always wanted to visit far places, see the lands that lie beyond the sun, yet I felt I had no choice but to stay in England and be a responsible heir. Then...someone made me realize I had all of the choices in the world. It's time to do what I've always yearned to do."

Dominic held out his hand to his brother. "Just remember to come home someday."

Kyle clasped his hand hard. "I shall."

Their gazes met, and Dominic's distress began to ease. Even with half a world between them, they would not be as separated as they had in the past.

"I'm giving you Pegasus. When you ride him, think of me." Struggling to control his expression, Kyle turned and moved into the crowd just as the church doors opened. The bridal couple emerged, laughing, and Meriel joined Dominic in time to toss handfuls of white rose petals at Lucia and her beaming new husband. At least someone in the family knew how to have a normal courtship and wedding, Dominic thought wryly as he threw the last of the fragrant petals.

Custom satisfied, Meriel seized Dominic's hand and led him around the church to the far end of the churchyard. "Come look!" She stopped by a clump of blue flowers. "I've never seen these before. Do you think the vicar will allow me to take some specimens back to Warfield?"

The blossoms looked unremarkable to Dominic, but Meriel was the expert. "I should think so. We'll come back tomorrow and ask." He glanced around and saw that there was no one else in sight, so he drew her close. "I haven't kissed you since we left Dornleigh to come to the church."

"I knew it seemed like a very long time," she said demurely.

Her kiss had the rapturous honesty that held nothing back. Breathing quickened and hands roamed until her back was pressed against a tree, his body pinning hers with the greatest intimacy achievable while still dressed.

Breathless with passion and laughter, Meriel tilted back her head. "I suppose you're going to tell me that it really won't do to make love under an oak at your sister's wedding when anyone might come around the church at any moment."

Reluctantly he stepped back. "You took the words out of my mouth. But think of how much anticipation will add to fulfillment when we are finally alone together."

"I'm thinking, I'm thinking," she murmured, expression sultry.

As she straightened her gown, he said abruptly, "Kyle's leaving England indefinitely. To see the world."

Her gaze met his. "I'm sorry. You must be far sorrier."

"Yes, but I'll survive. I'm glad he'll be doing what he has always wanted." He put an arm around her shoulders. "Let's walk back to Dornleigh for the wedding breakfast rather than take one of the carriages."

She nodded, and they ambled through the back gate onto the wooded path that would eventually take them to the great house. As they entered a cool tunnel of trees, Dominic said, "Kyle mentioned that my father wants to petition the Crown to have the Grahame title transferred to you and me rather than become dormant. Would you like to be Lady Grahame?"

She thought for the space of a dozen steps, then slanted him an intimate smile. "I should like to see our son, when we have one, carry the title borne by you and my father."

Joy bubbled through him as he realized that she was no longer uneasy about the prospect of children. A wife, the land, a family. What more could any man want? "Have I mentioned lately how much I love you?"

"Not in at least an hour. Far, far too long. Now it's my turn. I love you, Dominic, body and soul." Smiling mischievously, she went into his arms and rubbed against him sensually. "Most definitely with my body."

His blood caught fire again. As he kissed her, he realized that this path was far more private than the churchyard....

Mary Jo Putney was born in upstate New York. After earning degrees in English literature and industrial design at Syracuse University, she did various forms of design work in California and England before moving to Baltimore, Maryland, where she has lived very comfortably ever since.

In 1987, she gave up her freelance graphic design business to become a full-time writer. To date she has published twenty books, including *The Rake and the Reformer*, *Dancing on the Wind*, *River of Fire*, *Silk and Secrets*, and the national bestseller *One Perfect Rose*. She has won numerous writing awards, including two RITAs from the Romance Writers of America and several *Romantic Times* Awards.

She is currently at work on her next historical romance, *The China Bride*.